AGELESS BEAUTY

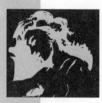

A Dermatologist's

Secrets for

Looking Younger

Without Surgery

AGELESS
BEAUTY

STEVEN VICTOR, M.D., and INA YALOF

Crown Publishers • New York

To my patients and to my beautiful daughters,
Andrea and Allison

Published by Crown Publishers, New York, New York.
Member of the Crown Publishing Group, a division of Random House, Inc.
www.randomhouse.com

CROWN is a trademark and the Crown colophon is a registered trademark of Random House, Inc.

Printed in the United States of America

DESIGNED BY ELINA D. NUDELMAN

Library of Congress Cataloging-in-Publication Data

Victor, Steven.

   Ageless beauty : a dermatologist's secrets for looking younger without surgery / Steven Victor and Ina Yalof.—1st ed.

   1. Skin—Care and hygiene.   2. Beauty, Personal.

   1. Cosmetic Techniques—Popular Works.   2. Skin Aging—Popular Works. WR 650 V645a 2003]   I. Yalof, Ina L., 1939–   II. Title.

   RL87.V53   2003

   646.7'26—dc21   2002006531

ISBN 0-8129-3219-6

10 9 8 7 6 5 4 3 2 1

First Edition

ACKNOWLEDGMENTS

I want to thank my mother, Bernice Victor, for encouraging my early love of medicine and ultimately of dermatology. For sustaining that interest and for their guidance throughout my career, I am eternally grateful to my mentors, Drs. Samuel Peck, Leo Orris, Norman Orentreich, and Victor Selmanowitz. My staff—and Monika Krasuska in particular—have been a great help throughout the writing of this book. It would not have been possible without them. I would also like to thank my wife, Anna Rhodes-Victor, for her love and support.

Gratitude is offered to Kim Witherspoon, my agent, for her unfailing guidance and for bringing me together with my savvy coauthor, Ina Yalof. Ina never missed a Wednesday afternoon meeting and kept me on the straight and narrow throughout. She did an outstanding job of guiding me through the joys (and frustration) of book writing and book publishing, and I am actually ready to do this again.

Contents

The Wrinkling of America

We're living in an incredible era. For the first time in human history, we can minimize or totally obliterate the outward signs of aging. Years' worth of "character lines" can be eradicated in a matter of minutes. Fifty-year-olds are mistaken for forty, and *forty* looks *thirty*. Today we have at our fingertips an arsenal of scientifically sanctioned treatments and products to slow the process of skin aging. Better still, we can even reverse its perceptible signs. It's all here for the taking: Botox to bronzers, collagen to cellulite massage. And why *shouldn't* we take full advantage of what science has to offer? After all, we bike and hike, we sweat and steam, we eat daily diets of macro and micro. We feel great!

So why not *look* that way, too?

Ladies and gentlemen, it is no secret: an aging epidemic is upon us. Only 25 years ago the average combined life expectancy for men and women in the United States was

71.4 years. Today, thanks as much to modern medicine as to our own commitment to healthy living, we can expect to enjoy our lives into our eighties, nineties, and beyond. People over 65 account for well over 12 percent of the American population (a figure that is expected to double in about 30 years, when half the population will be over 50), with people over 85 making up the fastest-growing segment. And some admittedly optimistic gerontologists think that, by the middle of the new century, an average life span of 120–150 is not inconceivable.

Of course, the news that we're living longer and healthier lives than ever before is very good indeed. For the skin, however, our longer life span offers a mixed blessing. For all of science's great strides toward improving our overall health, we are living in an ever-more-polluted and ozone-depleted world. And what absorbs the brunt of this environmental assault—of which ultraviolet damage is the main culprit? That vital organ called the skin.

These days we are vastly equipped to stave off some of the effects of our toxic atmosphere through better-formulated sunscreens and a better understanding of what causes our skin to become oxidized, denatured, and destroyed. But no advent of medicine can change the fact that the skin is an outer layer, the first line of defense that protects us from the outside world. So it hardly seems fair that, in the line of duty, it should "take it on the chin," so to speak. Long before its effects are even detected, time exacts an unforgiving toll on our appearance, making many of us unrecognizable even to ourselves. Who among us has not walked past a mirror or a store window and, after a furtive glance, thought, "What is my *mother* (or *father*) doing in there?" Although not all of us experience the aging process in the same way, no one would deny that its outward manifestations are proportional to our longevity. The longer we live, the older we're going to look.

For a long while medicine was considered a discipline for disease prevention and restoration and maintenance of health. Then, I admit, there wasn't much use for people like me. It is only recently that medicine, beset with an unprecedented number of patients seeking to reclaim their youthful looks, has come to grips with the aging of skin.

Maybe no one dies of wrinkles or age spots, but the austere notion that good looks don't matter comes as a poor consolation to those whose aging skin does not match their youthful soul. Let's not mince words. We've all learned from a very young age that good looks matter more than it is polite to admit. "Cute" babies get more attention than their less adorable brothers and sisters do. We don't need scientific studies to tell us (although there are many that do just that) that attractive people get more dates, land better jobs with higher salaries, and tend to be judged smarter, happier, more sociable, and more likely to be successful than their homelier peers. Furthermore, because interpersonal dynamics are by definition reciprocal—good-looking people draw positive responses from others, and those positive responses foster positive interaction in turn—a slightly embarrassing physical attribute, like a pimple, laugh lines, or liver spots, becomes far more embarrassing when you can't shake the feeling that someone you're talking to is staring right at it. True? You know it is.

Indeed, the importance placed on good looks in our culture, sad as it may sound, cannot be exaggerated. If you think that fact is stupid and frivolous and not worth worrying about, if you want to take the cosmetics and fashion industries to task for perpetuating the myth that beauty confers happiness, you may be right, and more power to you. But the reality is that appearance counts.

Ageless Beauty is aimed at helping you look your best *without surgery*. But you cannot look your best if you don't look natural. The only correct expectation of any cosmetic treatment, be it doctor-performed or over-the-counter, is a *realistic expectation*, pure and simple. I preach that message all day long. Many of my colleagues own a computer that allows them to take a picture of a person's face and morph it into the way it will look after certain cosmetic procedures. The reason I haven't used it is because I know I can't make those changes in real life. And so the patient is usually disappointed. I hate to show "before and after" pictures of my old patients because new patients will surely be disappointed in the end if they don't have the same results—and you can't have equal results if you don't start out with an equal canvas. A fifty-year-old woman will bring in a photo of Meg Ryan and say, "Make me look like this!" And indeed, I wish I could. I can't. I'm not sure anyone can.

Here's another situation: One of my patients recently had a deep laser treatment to her face and Botox to her forehead, and she looked great. No issue there. But six months later she came back, still looking great, and she said, "Do more. I want to look better than I look now." I explained to her that it's just not going to happen. I said, "You look terrific. I can't do any more to you. This is it." And she said, "In the last three months, I've gotten used to looking like this, and now I want to look even better." I still couldn't do it. There's a point at which you look as great as you can, and that's it. She actually had realistic expectations when I did her face, but she grew comfortable with the look and was disappointed that I wouldn't accommodate her further. I'm sure someone else did. I'm also sure that she was disappointed with the result, because if you overdo it, the patient loses his or her natural look and begins to look plastic.

Radical transformation is not impossible these days, but it's certainly not the rule. This is not to suggest—and I can't emphasize this enough—that there is nothing one can do, even in the grand scheme of things, to keep the signs of aging at bay. Quite the contrary. If there were no ways to make an aging face look astonishingly youthful again, I wouldn't be writing this book. Sure, I believe in aging gracefully like the next guy, but remember that the notion of aging gracefully has drastically changed in the past two decades. Just as people are continuing to live longer and healthier lives, shouldn't their skin share in that longevity and vitality? It seems to me, as a doctor as well as an avid follower of my own advice, the answer is clear.

In one sense your skin is no different from any other organ in your body. Yet no other part of you performs such vital bodily functions while also serving as a barrier against the outside world. The natural cycle of skin renewal seems simple: old skin cells are continually shed and replaced with new ones that float up from below the surface to take their place. These new cells actually produce skin as soft as a newborn baby's, skin that would remain that way were it not for external factors and environmental effects such as the sun and the wind.

Just nature alone can damage the newborn cells, causing them to grow irregularly. Even losing weight so that the stretched skin is no longer filled out has its effect. Nutritional factors, too, affect the growing cycle of the skin cell and, as we shall see in Chapter 12, can either help or hurt it. Add near-constant bombardment by ultraviolet light and other toxins to the equation and it becomes difficult for the skin to repair itself.

I'll save my ozone-layer diatribe for another day, but before reading any further, you must understand that intrinsic aging factors like sun and the pull of gravity are only part of what causes your skin to change. The other part involves the myriad uncontrollable genetic abnormalities that prematurely age the skin—the impaired blood-vessel function of diabetes, for example, or autoimmune-related skin disorders. But take heart. It's all "fixable" to a large degree. And soon we shall see how.

The wear and tear that skin endures affects different skin types differently, and although heredity still has a lot to do with it, aging signs vary significantly depending on your lifestyle. Even fair-skinned, natural blondes—the most susceptible to sun damage or "photoaging"—can, through prevention and self-care, defy the years. But I'm getting ahead of myself. First I want to draw the broad outlines of normal aging, so that you can know what to expect and what you can reverse.

Believe it or not, the effects of aging on the skin begin to show as early as our late twenties, when we notice just the slightest appearance of fine lines and wrinkles, especially around the eyes and above the upper lip—the consequence of a gradual, but steady, loss of moisture and elasticity. A few years further down the road, we observe those *nasolabial* (or, more euphemistically, "smile") lines, slight furrows in the forehead and folds between the eyes, an unmistakable loosening of the jowls and neck, and excess skin above the eyes.

Introduction

The reality is that, like clockwork, each decade will leave its own marks and deepen the effects of those before it. How deeply is determined by two variables: heredity and lifestyle. Heredity includes the variables of genes, skin color, bone structure, hormonal output. Lifestyle includes time spent in the sun (yes, your teen years count), smoking, exercise (which improves your vascularity and your skin's texture), skin color (the more pigment your skin houses, the more protected you are), and yo-yo dieting, in which your skin tends to stretch and relax, stretch and relax.

More bad news: With age our complexions get duller, brown spots begin to appear, and fatty pockets develop above and under the eyes and under the chin; our skin sweats less and produces less oil, steadily drying out and losing its luster. Postadolescent acne and other blemish disorders may also rear their ugly heads, fueled in part by hormone imbalances, which greet us later in life. A glance in a full-length mirror confirms that aging is not confined to the face. Spotted, thin-skinned hands are a dead giveaway, as are spider veins on the legs, thinning hair on our heads, and keratoses, which are rough growths on the skin, popping up like dandelions just about everywhere. These changes make us look older than we feel or feel older than we are—paradoxical conditions that I have always found immensely disquieting. But take heart. They, too, are treatable.

With an ever-expanding array of nonsurgical treatment options, the field of cosmetic dermatology has made staggering advances in the past two decades and continues to keep pace with the exponentially surging demand for aesthetic medicine. By now many of these procedures—such as chemical peeling, laser resurfacing, and collagen injections, to name the most common—have become firmly entrenched in the beauty vernacular. But there are other treatments, new, cutting-edge, not so well publicized. How many people know, for instance, that *mesotherapy*—the injection of a vitamin- and mineral-rich solution directly into the dermis—is far more effective at enriching the skin than the traditional patches and creams? How many people are aware that laser resurfacing, thanks to new low-heat lasers that can be set specifically for each patient's skin type, now means minimal recovery time and discomfort? These are but two tricks of the trade we'll discuss.

Now, of course, you may be wondering: Why choose these treatments over plastic surgery? Isn't plastic surgery still the way to go for truly transformative results? In most cases, the answer is a resounding *no*. Naturally there is an important place for plastic surgery, which, in fact, I recom- mend to patients as a worthy complement to certain resur- facing techniques, if I think it's merited. But no matter how old you are or how many wrinkles you have, if your skin isn't sagging, your first visit should absolutely, unequivo- cally be to a cosmetic dermatologist.

Plastic surgery can get the wrinkles out, no question, but below the surface things are pretty much the same. You will still have sun damage, and your collagen will still be in sad shape because your skin cells are turning over at the same dwindling rate. Let's face it: you can have your skin pulled, clipped, and tucked to no end, but if it's dull and blotchy, if it's not working any better beneath the epidermis to repair itself, it is not improving your skin's overall health. Many of the treatments I will describe have been proved as successful as plastic surgery in restoring the skin's youthful elasticity. So again, although you may in the end need surgery to get the optimum results, it's more than worth your while to see what a cosmetic dermatologist can do for you first.

This book is all about keeping your skin vital, healthy, and youthful year after year after year. By this I mean having skin that not only *looks* vital, healthy, and youthful but behaves that way as well. The procedures I will discuss can improve the vascularity of the skin by inducing the formation of new blood vessels (which, in turn, improves skin color and nutrition). These procedures can also stimulate cell turnover, eliminate the blotches or "dispigmentation" caused by accumulated melanin, and, yes, promote the growth of new dermal collagen. The result: smoother, clearer, firmer, radiant skin. Who doesn't want that?

In recent years, a number of books have outlined—some quite admirably—practical, at-home routines for preventing or reversing the signs of aging. The idea behind such books is that, through a carefully followed regimen of skin care, diet, vitamins and exercise, the need for surgery can, if you start young enough, be indefinitely forestalled. But does it really work for everyone? What about those people—and believe me, I've treated many of them—who, no matter how diligently they exercise, diet, or keep up a sensible skin routine, find the results of their hard work disappointing at best? For many people, particularly those who have spent much of their youth in the sun or who have inherited less resilient skin, the effects of a daily skin-care program can ultimately be underwhelming; for others the payoff, however substantial, is just too agonizingly slow. What sorts of procedures are out there for people who are committed to taking care of their skin but who also aren't satisfied with do-it-yourself therapies?

Funny you should ask. *Ageless Beauty* is a comprehensive guide to understanding what the newest procedures in non-surgical cosmetic enhancement can do to help people of all ages—across all skin types and colorations—turn back the clock. With this book I'll tell you about the new, formidable weapons against aging—in fact, a whole arsenal of treatments that will let you look as young and as good as you feel.

Beginning with the premise that it's never too late to correct skin damage, whatever the cause, or too early to start protecting against it (my own patients range from their twenties to their eighties), the battle plan proposed here is very simple and won't ask you to run out and buy a line of products you don't need.

The meat of the book is in Chapter 3, "At Face Value," which focuses on the myriad procedures that reverse the signs of aging, and not just on the face. This chapter goes into these procedures in depth, but many will be repeated in later chapters, though not in quite so much detail. Because the face is only part of the picture, I've included additional chapters on the care and treatment of the hair and scalp, the hands and the legs, even the teeth, all of which change as we age and transform our overall appearance. The chapter called "Gloves Off!" for instance, addresses, among other things, the treatments available to transform those telltale age-spotted, ropy-looking hands. "Crowning Glories" examines the latest procedures for slowing and/or stopping both male and female baldness, including an in-depth look at new hair-grafting techniques and *finasteride*—otherwise known as the "baldness pill."

Introduction

I've devoted a chapter to men, who age differently from women, physically and psychologically. Men's needs are addressed throughout the book, but in "For Men Only," I bring the male aging process into focus, examine the aging signs that men find most distressing, and detail what can be done about them. Although men are not as prone as women to expressing their concerns about wrinkles (any more than they're prone to asking directions when they're lost), they do care about looking as youthful and vital as possible. Vain, fragile creatures that we are, how could they not? We all know that men have always been obsessed with their physiques, and it is becoming increasingly apparent that that concern extends even to facial aging, which, no less than hair loss, has an insidious way of detracting from all the hard work a guy puts in at the gym. Although men, as far as I can tell, are not yet swapping beauty secrets at the makeup counter, the male cosmetics industry is booming; men in unprecedented numbers are wearing sunscreen and buying up wrinkle remedies packaged as shaving creams and other "acceptable" formulations. Topping it all off, you will read a chapter on food and vitamins and how you can make them work for you as partners in your quest for perfect skin texture and tone.

The House We Live In

Ever since people like me set out to explain this wondrous human garment known as the skin, analogies have abounded. "The skin is like a glove, constantly subjected to earth, wind, and fire and twisted this way and that." "The skin is like a pair of leggings, fitting you snugly until one day it bunches up and begins to sag." "The skin is like a piece of paper on which your whole life story is written overnight."

Indeed, each of these comparisons carries its own metaphorical weight; each helps us understand the skin's capacity to protect and break down, to be a window onto our beauty and, suddenly, a ledger of our years. And yet there seems to me something decidedly inadequate about comparing the skin to some formfitting garment or gift wrap, as if it were something to be unsheathed and tossed away when it is no longer presentable.

To be sure, the skin is thin, not to say flimsy. All told, it's about eighteen-thousandths of an inch thick, give or take a few thousandths. But it's a major working organ as well, the largest organ in our body, in fact. The skin is charged with several roles: preventing the leakage of vital fluids into the environment, regulating the body's temperature, responding to sensations, excreting wastes, absorbing nutrients, even producing vitamin D. Even more crucially, it acts as a protective barrier against bacteria, ultraviolet rays, the environment, and other assailants—keeping us in one piece, so to speak. The importance of this latter function becomes especially apparent when the top layer of the skin is lost, as in the case of a third-degree burn, leaving the tissues beneath exposed to the environment and thus highly susceptible to damage and disease.

All of which brings me to my own preferred metaphor: *the house*. Yes, this metaphor is bulkier, clumsier, even, how shall I say, homelier. But it is the only one I can think of that appropriately conveys the complexity and substance of this vital organ, not to mention the constant, unstinting care that is needed to keep it in "working order." More than a *twenty-square-foot, seven to ten-pound bodily shield*, the skin is vastly expressive, variously blushing, bristling, and blanching with embarrassment, aggravation, and horror. This brings me to the distinction between social skin and biological skin that my field has been considering for decades. As I have suggested, the skin manages to perform its biological functions extraordinarily well, even as time plays havoc with its surface. Similarly a well-built house may be no less cozy or efficient even when badly in need of a fresh coat of paint.

Still—and all you homeowners will know what I mean here—if you don't keep a house up, it falls into disrepair before you turn around, and eventually it becomes twice as hard to return it to its original, beautiful state. Accordingly we may be lucky with our analogy here, because while houses don't repair themselves, nature has seen to it that the skin does, at least for a while, anyway. But then, as time goes on, even cells wear out.

How, then, does this deterioration occur? What accounts for the body's gradual inability, at the molecular level, to repair itself by replacing its worn-out cells with new ones? Dozens of aging theories have been posited over the years, and science still has not yet pinned down a single, unified understanding of how we grow old. While the "neuroendocrine theory," for example, attributes aging symptoms to dwindling hormone levels and thus points to hormone replacement therapy as a possible biochemical fountain of youth, the "wear-and-tear" theory offers the undeniable view that cells, no matter how carefully preserved, cannot long endure the daily abuse that is "living."

Every theory out there more or less centers on an idea that lies at the very heart of cellular biology: aging is a mechanism, encoded within our DNA, without which our species could not feasibly survive. In other words, cells, whose self-replication is the essence of human life, are also programmed to sustain the life of the human race by shutting down when necessary. Of course, the biological clock that determines the life span of cells is affected greatly by how we choose to live, but the bottom line is that cells can turn over only so many times before they can no longer function. A fairly recently observed phenomenon known as *telomere shortening* in fact guarantees as much. Every time a fresh cell carrying the same genetic data replaces a worn-out cell, the *telomere,* a protein responsible for maintaining the integrity of chromosomes, is shortened, leading to cellular damage and death. However, this process has also led to an uplifting discovery. In 2000, scientists figured out a way to trigger the cellular production of *telomerase,* an enzyme found in germ and cancer cells that maintains telomere length. Telomerase appears to dramatically alter the life span of dividing cells and may even, theoretically, "immortalize" them. It is also believed that skin cells would respond especially well to this sort of chromosome manipulation—which, believe it or not, may be performed within this decade.

All the more reason to take care of yourself in the meantime—to take advantage of today's antiaging remedies, and there are many, so that when measures like gene therapy arrive, there will be little to reverse. This is especially true for the skin, the outward appearance of which, as with any "house," is invariably a reflection of inner health, stability, and longevity.

So, how to do this? Actually, as this book will show you, it's quite simple. Stay out of the sun whenever possible and use sunscreen, no matter what your skin color or type. Don't smoke. Keep your weight as constant as possible. Exfoliate regularly with alpha hydroxy acids and, under a dermatologist's supervision, Retin-A. Eat well, focusing on minimizing the production of free radicals. Understand that the best way to avoid skin damage is to stop doing your skin harm.

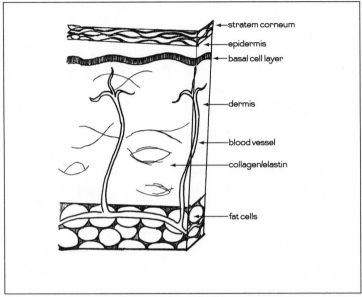

Diagram of Skin

And finally, when intervention is required to reverse the changes brought on by the years, familiarize yourself with every realistic and safe treatment option, surgical and non-surgical alike.

THE STRUCTURE OF THE SKIN

Let's now turn briefly to the structure of the skin. The skin is made up of two essential layers, the dermis and the epidermis, each of which breaks down differently over time. The top layer of the two, the extremely thin epidermis (which is thickest on the palms and soles), is itself composed of two layers—the living basal layer and the outer coat of packed dead (or "keratinized") cells called the *stratum corneum*. The stratum corneum is shed regularly by younger skin as the basal layer produces a near-constant flow of keratinocytes, which float up and replace worn-out cells at the surface. The stratum is the layer on which we are all so fixated. It blotches, blemishes, burns, dries up, and, yes, wrinkles; it manifests all the damage done to the lower layers and even to the upper layers when the basal layer's capacity for producing fresh cells slows with age. Below it the epidermis also contains *melanocytes*, the melanin-producing cells that determine our skin color—and our susceptibility to sun damage. With some notable exceptions I will discuss later, the more skin-darkening melanin our skin produces, the greater its protection against ultraviolet rays.

Think of the epidermis as the body's paint and shingles, a protective coating that itself requires a great deal of protection from the environment. The dermis is the skin's underlying framework, the crucial connective layer whose tissue contains the blood vessels, lymph channels, nerve endings, glands that secrete perspiration and sebum (oil), and hair follicles—all the things, in other words, that make the skin an active organ. The function of your oil glands, for instance, is to prevent the skin and hair from drying out; dry skin tends to crack more easily, creating potential inlets for bacteria.

When the body is overheated, the sweat glands in the dermis secrete water onto the skin's surface, where it evaporates and cools the body, while blood vessels in the dermis called arterioles dilate, increasing blood flow through the dermis and bringing excess heat close to the skin surface to be radiated into the environment. When the body is cold, sweat glands don't secrete, and the arterioles constrict to keep heat from being lost. In other words, your dermis connects your skin to a host of vital functions that keep you alive and well.

The uneven nexus between the epidermis and dermis is called the *papillary layer*, where an abundance of capillaries exists to nourish the cell-generating *basal layer*, which has no blood supply of its own. Just beneath that junction, the substance within the dermis that harbors all of its vital structures is primarily that all-consuming protein known as *collagen*. Generated by cells called *fibroblasts*, collagen is a strong protein fiber organized in a series of parallel microscopic bands—an arrangement that affords it great strength and flexibility. Combined with a more flexible substance called *elastin* that resides within it, collagen determines how well the skin fits and how much stretching it can withstand. It is thicker in men than in women. When it becomes weakened, either through sun exposure or through the repetitive stress of, say, squinting or pursing the lips around a cigarette, it loses elasticity and breaks down, causing our skin to sag. Around the eyes, for example, the repeated contractions of the *orbis oculi muscle* that occur when you smile or squint in effect etch lines into the area—almost like crinkling a sheet of paper—by stretching out the collagen below. Collagen breakdown is a major source of wrinkles, in other words, and as I will show you, there is so much that we can do nowadays to keep your collagen healthy and resilient.

Below the collagen, finally, our "house" finds its foundation. The layer of fat and, below that, muscle on which the skin is poised is similar to a house's substructure, an extremely solid yet thoroughly supple groundwork, both shock-absorbent and sturdy. In addition to storing excess nutrients and providing insulation from the cold, the fatty tissue beneath the skin conceals wrinkles by keeping the skin plump and filled out. The loss of subcutaneous fat with age, particularly around the mouth, is one of the more paradoxical causes of wrinkles, but it is definitely one of the most troublesome; and while I caution against obesity, I never hesitate to warn my patients of the dermatological dangers of being too thin. Similarly it is vitally important to keep your underlying muscles firm but not overtaxed. Remember that muscles, like collagen, are elastic, and high-impact exercises like running (or those facial exercises you once heard about) can do more harm than good.

Before I go on to review what changes the years bring, I want to reemphasize that there is no single determinant of aging effects, that many, many factors accelerate the inexorable wear and tear we all, at some basic level, must accept. Heredity (the "pure luck" factor that determines texture, tone, and indeed, the very longevity of our skin); sun exposure; our propensity (or lack thereof) for losing or gaining unhealthy amounts of weight; the slightest, most innocuous-seeming personal habits (squinting hourly at a distant clock, tugging at your chin)—all of these are part of the equation. Fortunately we now have the tools at hand to keep most of their consequences at bay.

two

The Ages of Aging

A friend of Dorothy Parker's once remarked that she hated to think of life at forty, to which that mordant wit replied, "Why? What happened then?"

I expect your friends are kinder and less candid than Dorothy Parker was, but not so your mirror. You can always count on it to tell you the truth. That's the thing about mirrors—day by day they tend to reflect the face you've inherited and unflinchingly herald its hike across the years.

Happily we have many ways to correct some of nature's mistakes—and our own. But before we consider them, let's look at what happens to our skin over the decades, bearing in mind, if you will, that this is only an approximate guide. Certain skin changes may overlap two decades. It's important to factor in, too, that each of us is unique; we all age at different rates and in varying degrees. In my own practice, I see twenty-year-old sun worshipers who appear much older and fifty- and sixty-year-olds with good genes who appear much younger.

THE TWENTIES

Then come kiss me, sweet and twenty,
Youth's a stuff will not endure.

—Shakespeare, *Twelfth Night*

Twenty is sweet, indeed, although our skin has already suffered some damage below the surface. Women usually don't begin to detect any true signs of aging until their mid- to late twenties (or even their early thirties), when pronounced changes in the skin and its underlying structures take place. This shift tends to occur about five to seven years later in men, whose skin is thicker due to thicker hair follicles. When it comes to aging effects, blondes definitely do *not* have more fun: olive- or black-skinned brunettes with dark eyes commonly age more slowly (by five to ten years) than their fair-complexioned, blue-eyed sisters.

At some point in our twenties, important cellular changes begin. The stratum corneum starts to thicken. This takes away some of that youthful glow, replacing it with a duller, ruddier look. In the meantime the metabolism of the basal-cell layer (the bottom layer of the epidermis) gradually slows, which further thins the epidermis. These alterations in the cellular mechanism also cause the skin to lose its ability to retain moisture. The combination of all these phenomena makes the skin vulnerable to wrinkles.

Fine lines appear first around the eyes, where the skin is thinnest and most delicate, and above the upper lip. These two areas especially reflect our vacillating facial expressions, like smiling, frowning, grimacing, and squinting. The faint lines we see at the corners of our eyes are harbingers of the deeper, more noticeable crow's-feet to come later. When pursing our lips in the mirror, as if for a kiss, we may see the beginning of vertical pleating right above them. Smokers will usually develop these particular lines before nonsmokers. (Look in the mirror as you inhale that next cigarette, and I promise you'll discover yet another reason to quit.)

Estrogen protects women's hair from any major changes during their twenties. Men with inherited balding patterns, however, may notice some thinning. The skin of the chest, back, hands, and legs does not generally show changes yet, either, although spider veins may begin to appear on some women's legs.

THE THIRTIES

I swear she's no chicken; she's
on the wrong side of thirty, if she be a day.

—Jonathan Swift, *Polite Conversation*

When the TV series *thirtysomething* aired, people of all ages and stripes identified with that wonderful decade of life—when we're old enough to have absorbed a little wisdom, and young enough to use it. Many of my older patients recall looking their best during their thirties, but nowadays even thirtysomethings will detect slight changes in their skin they don't like. Those fine lines they first noticed in their twenties are definitely deepening, and others, between the eyes (the global area) and from the nose to the mouth (nasolabial, or "laugh," lines), are becoming visible. This is largely the result of damage to collagen and elastin in the dermis. A thirty-year-old smiling broadly in the mirror can see several of the coming attractions (or detractions) of aging.

Estrogen continues to protect a woman's hair and, in many respects, her skin, but the skin tends to be slightly drier. And dreaded cellulite may begin, with fine dimpling on the sides and backs of the thighs. The veins of the hands become slightly more prominent, due to the hands' gradually thinning skin and a slight loss of underlying fat. More spider veins may appear, especially behind the knees.

For most men changes up to this point—unless they have included hair loss—have been hardly noticeable. Now marked changes are taking place, particularly to the thin skin around the eyes, which years of squinting, smiling, and sun have creased, and in the nasolabial fold. Men's skin also tends to loosen at this point, producing bags under the eyes and in some cases loose flesh beneath the chin. Although these changes do not seem to be disturbing to most, they bother more men than ever before.

THE FORTIES

I am resolved to grow fat and look young
till forty, and then slip out of the world
with the first wrinkle and the
reputation of five-and-twenty.

—John Dryden, *The Maiden Queen*

Life doesn't really begin at forty, as the saying goes, but it's hardly over then, either. And because of all the advances in cosmetic dermatology, the long-held belief that a woman in early middle age has to choose between her face and her figure is no longer true. You don't have to "grow fat" to continue looking young in your visage, although the loss of fatty tissue under our skin contributes greatly to that "first wrinkle" and all the others that follow.

In our forties, whether we're fat or thin, our jowls and neck start to loosen and sag. This happens because the collagen and elastin fibers of the dermis become less organized and weaker. In addition, the layer of fat beneath it decreases, and the muscle structure begins to break down. There may be a dilation of a few blood vessels in the face (erroneously referred to as "broken" blood vessels), making them visible. The veins of the hands become more prominent, and "liver" spots (which have nothing to do with your liver) begin to appear, especially in fair-skinned people and those who've experienced excessive sun exposure. Cellulite also becomes more prominent in our forties. The dimpling on the sides and backs of the thighs deepens a bit, and cellulite begins to appear on the buttocks.

Another fortyish complaint comes from patients who seem to be revisiting the worst part of their adolescence: yes, acne! "I wanted to be young again," a forty-three-year-old woman recently complained, "but this wasn't what I meant." Others, who were blessed with clear skin in their teens, are dismayed to find themselves breaking out for the first time twenty years later. To make things worse, adult-onset acne manifests itself in painful and deep-seated cysts rather than the more superficial teenage "zits." Adult acne commonly appears on the sides of the face and around the jawline and chin, as opposed to the more centralized teenage acne, and unlike teenage acne, it often continues into old age. What happens is this: Stress causes the pituitary gland to stimulate the adrenal glands, which then produce androgens. These androgens stimulate the oil glands, which cause acne to break out.

Men in their mid- to late forties are (finally!) beginning to see dramatic, distressing changes. In lighter-skinned men who have suffered a lot of sun exposure, this will mean a sudden proliferation of deep lines, grooves, and wrinkles— seemingly sudden, I should say, for the damage has been accumulating for years. In men with darker skin, the skin will loosen and sag more than wrinkle, but the psychic effect is the same. The frown line between the eyes and nasolabial grooves on either side of the mouth begin to look deeply etched, and crow's-feet around the eyes are pronounced; eyelid skin is loose, and puffy bags below the eyes are very common. The bearded areas of the face are still quite youthful due to thicker hair follicles and shaving, which effectively exfoliates the skin.

THE FIFTIES

Love is lame at fifty years.

—Thomas Hardy, "The Revisitation"

Maybe love was pretty lame at fifty in Hardy's time. After all, when he died, in 1928, the average life span in the United States was only 54.6 years. Conspicuous new skin changes may be observed during our fifties as earlier ones continue to become more pronounced.

You may not think it's a pretty picture, but I remind you that there are many ways to deal with it. By this time the stratum corneum has thickened significantly, the epidermis has thinned much more, and the cellular metabolic rate is way down. The collagen and elastin fibers are now so disorganized and weak that the skin begins to stretch, leaving it prey to gravity. Among other effects, this can result in what we perceive as "fallen" eyebrows and "masked" cheekbones. Just about everywhere, from the upper lip to the corners of the eyes, fine lines don't look fine at all. Blotches and age spots are plain as day. And the fat layer around the mouth has thinned so much; there is sometimes a caved-in look that draws the corners of the mouth downward. The skin of the upper and lower eyelids is stretched to excess, and frown lines between the eyebrows no longer snap back as they used to. Overall there is a loss of youthful fullness in the face, hands, neck, and lips. It becomes difficult for many women to apply lipstick, because the lip line has begun to grow less distinct.

In our early fifties the sebaceous/oil glands become less productive, causing dryness in the skin, hair, and nails; and the onset of menopause lowers the estrogen supply, allowing inherited male-pattern baldness in some women to begin. At the same time, the skin on their backs may become thicker, and the skin on their chests starts to crinkle.

Men, too, are suffering most of these changes; by now their age has fully caught up with them, even if they believe they still look twenty-one. Excess skin in the eyelids, bags below the eyes, smile lines, a loosening of the brow that pushes the eyebrows downward, drooping jowls, a thick nasolabial fold—men in their fifties are going through the worst of it. On the plus side, hair loss generally stops around the midfifties, so if you're still "holding strong" up top, you probably won't ever go bald.

THE SIXTIES

Will you still need me, will you still feed me,
When I'm 64?

—The Beatles, "When I'm 64"

Our grandmothers, in their sixties, usually dressed the part. (I remember my own grandmother wearing a Hoover apron over a shapeless housedress, that generation's notion of "the layered look." From the white-haired bun on her head to the bristly hairs on her chin, from her matronly posture to her orthopedic shoes, Grandma was just a sweet little old lady who seemed to live in the kitchen. Even when Grandpa was still alive, we never saw either of them—God forbid—as sexual beings.)

All that has changed, of course. Today's Grandma is a

senator, a doctor, a lawyer, a model, or a pilot. And if Grandpa still has his senses about him, he's probably chasing her around the bedroom. Chances are, she dresses for comfort and beauty from head to toe. Her hairdo is stylish, her posture is great, and the hairs on her chin are regularly plucked or waxed (alas, only temporary solutions). The thing is, people are not so easily thrown into age-determined categories anymore. The workforce has grown older, along with the general population, and we all want to look and feel our best.

During our sixties, though, a host of radical skin changes take place. There's a cross-hatching of wrinkles now in the cheeks. Secondary lines around the mouth actually extend below the jawline, creating the "marionette" effect, and keratoses, those rough little growths, appear in various places on the face and body. The oil glands of the face may become enlarged and visible (as little bumps), in their effort to compensate for lowered oil production, while previous wrinkles and loose skin grow more pronounced than ever. The upper eyelids will appear hooded, the lower lids wrinkled and loose, and the cheekbones less discernible. In addition, a horizontal line forms on the bridge of the nose, and another one appears above the lip. The nose gets slightly longer during this period, and the earlobes lengthen, too, become thinner, and develop wrinkles. Vertical pleats appear in front of the ears, and the skin on the chin tends to become "crepy." A further lowering of estrogen allows further hair thinning. Cellulite, spider veins, and the veins and age spots on the hands all become more prominent. The sixties may be the most traumatic decade, in terms of aging, a time when we look in the mirror and see our own mothers (or fathers) there.

THE SEVENTIES AND BEYOND

To be seventy years young is sometimes
more cheerful and hopeful than to be forty years old.

—Oliver Wendell Holmes, on the seventieth birthday
of Julia Ward Howe

By now it's no surprise that all the aging effects of the previous decades persist and deepen as we get older and older. Some seventysomethings may even look wistfully back at their sixty-year-old selves. However, you must understand that the extent to which time takes its toll will depend on you. If you spend your life ignoring the process, you won't be surprised to see the same changes getting worse. If, however, you've done everything possible to retain your vitality and good looks, seeking medical intervention where necessary and effective, you'll be pleasantly surprised to find that you look a lot younger than you are.

If that interests you, read on.

three

At Face Value

The face. This is where it all happens, folks, the core of our cosmetic universe. More than a decade has gone by since Linda Perney wryly observed in the magazine *Mirabella,* "In an era when surgeons rearrange skin and bones as casually as furniture—when one looks at a model and wonders if those are her own lips, breasts, chin—most women have at least thought about having something done." If that sounds like the start of an indictment, it wasn't meant to be. On the contrary, her article went on to discuss the benefits and pitfalls of a number of dermatological procedures that, about a decade ago, were taking the country by storm. "The key is to match the procedure to the problem," she cautioned, and that advice still applies today, when skin-care routines and medical treatments are recognized as virtually complementary practices. Provided that your expectations are realistic, that you don't believe you will emerge

At Face Value

from a procedure looking like a teenager again, that you don't expect to eliminate every last wrinkle or fold, and that you opt for a treatment that works for your problem, *there's very little skin damage that you have to live with.*

Nonsurgical antiaging treatments fall into two equally popular camps: resurfacing and fillers. Resurfacing uses chemicals, lasers, and other tools to remove wrinkled, damaged, or blemished skin so it can be replaced with a smoother, more lustrous version. Fillers encompass techniques that involve injecting under the skin foreign substances such as collagen to plump it up and/or otherwise restore the skin below the surface. As with any medical procedure, each of these options entails some degree of risk, but on the whole the medical and aesthetic risks are quite manageable. With laser resurfacing and chemical peels, for instance, there has always been some risk of discoloration (a contrast in skin tone between the treated and untreated areas), in darker-skinned patients especially, but these days our ability to individualize and fine-tune the peeling process is exceptional. All in all, while expectation must be carefully weighed against risk before undergoing any cosmetic treatment, the options listed below are as safe as they are remarkably effective.

RESURFACING PROCEDURES

Resurfacing the skin is essentially a matter of "off with the old—welcome to the new." Much of the skin's top layer is composed of dead and dying cells, which can cause a dull-looking complexion. When you exfoliate that layer, that is, when you peel it off, you send a message down to the

growing layers of skin to wake them up and get them producing new (and gorgeous) skin cells. This mechanism of
growing new skin by exfoliating the old was identified when,
in 1974, an interesting study was done with Scotch tape. The
research scientists literally removed the outer layer of the
subject's skin by pasting a strip of Scotch tape on the skin and
pulling it off many times over. Each time they did it, they got
a coating of cells. Eventually they got a complete layer of
skin. Then they did biopsies, and they studied the skin under
the microscope. They found that just by removing the outer
layer of skin, a signal was sent down to the growing layer of
skin beneath it saying, "OK, guys, wake up. Get busy. Generate a new layer of skin." So the new skin arrived, and when
it did, it looked younger than the skin it replaced.

Again, resurfacing procedures can be divided into two
types: topical and mechanical. Topical resurfacing is used
for milder symptoms of aging such as fine wrinkles and
age spots. These include chemical peels and prescription
drugs like Retin-A and bleaches or cosmetics containing
alpha and beta hydroxies, which are discussed further in
Chapter 10, "Preventions and Inventions." Mechanical resurfacing includes laser procedures and dermabrasion. These
treatments can go deeper and are, especially in the case of
dermabrasion, used to treat deeper scars and wrinkles.

Topical Resurfacing

TRETINOIN (RETIN-A AND RENOVA)

I'm certain most of you are familiar with Retin-A (the
generic name of which is tretinoin or retinoic acid). This
astonishing compound was created as a treatment for acne

in 1969 by pioneering dermatologist Dr. Albert Kligman
and his colleagues at the University of Pennsylvania School
of Medicine. And many of you may even recall the excite-
ment that seized the cosmetics world when, nearly twenty
years later, Dr. John Voorhees discovered that Retin-A could
work miracles on more than just acne. Here's what Vorhees
found: by the same process through which the vitamin
A–derived formula spurred cell turnover to expel the blackheads and whiteheads from which pimples develop, evidence
showed that Retin-A also *reversed* skin damage and significantly enhanced the skin's ability to renew itself. Indeed,
numerous studies (some of them admittedly funded by the
drug's manufacturer, the Ortho Pharmaceutical Corporation of Johnson & Johnson) have since demonstrated that
skin treated with topical retinoids shows a host of structural improvements, including the diminishment of fine
wrinkles, new blood vessel formation, and even an enhanced
ability to generate new bands of collagen within the dermis.
By increasing cell turnover, Retin-A causes *keratinocytes* to
move more quickly to the skin surface, a process that
improves the texture of the stratum corneum (the skin's
outermost layer) and helps to break up spotty discoloration.

How much truth is there to these dazzling claims? A
great deal, it turns out, although the exact extent of the
drug's efficacy is still a source of some dispute. And that's
because it doesn't work for everyone. Many men and women
who have since given up on the drug claim Retin-A has
failed to do much more than make their skin irritated, flaky,
and dry. Results tend to vary depending on whether it is
being used for wrinkles, age spots, or rough skin, but on the
whole a significant majority of tretinoin users report only

minimal improvement or none at all. *That is not, however, because the cream doesn't work.* Rather, it's because you must use it for eight to twelve weeks to see results, and most people don't want to deal with the flaking and irritation it takes to get to positive results. So they discontinue use after a very short while. Still, dissatisfied customers notwithstanding, the drug has proved remarkably effective in so many instances that there's simply no denying its promise.

What's the difference between Retin-A and Renova? Retin-A and Renova are made by the same manufacturer, Ortho Dermatological, and use the same active ingredient, tretinoin, in varying concentrations. The difference is that Renova is a rich emollient cream designed specifically to treat wrinkles, brown spots, and skin texture. It is less irritating than Retin-A and increasingly preferred by dermatologists for treating aging symptoms. Retin-A is still the chosen medication for acne.

Ortho is careful in its advertisements for Retin-A and Renova (both creams require a physician's prescription) to say that while tretinoin "will *not* eliminate wrinkles, repair sun damaged skin or reverse the aging process, it is proven to *reduce* fine wrinkles, *fade* brown spots, and *smooth* roughness." But this is only a disclaimer, designed to keep your expectations in check. In my experience, for every patient who uses Retin-A for several months and shows no improvement, there is another who has clearly benefited to some degree. Most dermatologists I know are fully behind the FDA's decision, in 1996, to make Renova, a relatively new formulation of Retin-A in a less irritating emollient base, the first drug ever approved by the government as a wrinkle remedy. It may not work for everyone, but it's absolutely worth a shot.

In any case, the truth is that even if Retin-A doesn't work wonders on existing wrinkles or firm up sagging skin, it will still dramatically improve the health of your skin and very probably forestall future wrinkles and folds. Not bad. What sets Retin-A apart from other exfoliants is that, unlike alpha hydroxy acids, which work on the skin's upper layers, tretinoin penetrates deep inside your skin, not only stimulating cell turnover but also prompting the basal layer to produce healthier, more "youthful" cells. In other words, it has a measurably positive influence on both the formation and shedding of skin cells and, if used correctly, can reverse or prevent sun damage that may soon result in wrinkles. However, because Retin-A works in part by inducing the skin to heal itself through controlled irritation, it can make the skin red and scaly during treatment and in all cases extremely sensitive to sun exposure. *You should be wearing an SPF 15 sunscreen with UVA and UVB protection every day anyway, but when using Renova or Retin-A, it is absolutely vital.*

Retin-A and Renova are serious medications and—for now, at least—available only by prescription. Your dermatologist should be keeping track of your progress while you are undergoing tretinoin therapy. Retin-A comes in a gel, liquid, or cream base. The best tolerated appears to be the .025 percent cream. Because tretinoin is intensely sun-sensitizing, it is applied nightly, before bedtime, twenty minutes after the skin has been properly cleansed with a mild soap and gently towel-dried. If you have sensitive skin, your doctor may have you start your therapy by applying it every other night. With Renova, a .05 percent tretinoin formulation in a rich emollient base, there is a far lower incidence of irritation, and doctors everywhere are beginning to prefer it to Retin-A.

How to Use Retin-A/Renova

To apply Renova, squeeze out a pea-sized amount on your fingertip and carefully spread it over your entire face. With Retin-A it takes about a half inch of cream to do the job. Be careful to keep it well away from your eyes, ears, nostrils, or mouth, which are too sensitive to handle retinoic acid. When you're done, the cream should be invisible; if it isn't, you're using too much, which only wastes medication and doesn't produce faster results. Both medications may sting or feel warm for a few seconds after application, and both may result in some redness and irritation, which, in most cases, soon subsides. If redness, flakiness, or irritation seriously persists with both Retin-A and Renova, however, your doctor may advise you to discontinue tretinoin therapy.

The morning after using tretinoin, it is essential to apply a moisturizer and sunscreen (I'm partial to keeping moisturizers and sunscreens separate, but moisturizers containing sunscreen save a step and are also quite effective) about thirty minutes before going outside. This gives the sunscreen ample time to be absorbed and protect your skin from sun exposure—which should be kept to a minimum. You may apply cosmetics in the meantime. Avoid products containing alcohol, spices, citrus, and other ingredients that may irritate the skin.

Results

With Renova or Retin-A, results may be seen in as soon as three to four months, but as a rule the drug's effects can be fairly assessed at the six-month point. Tretinoin at night can be used in tandem with alpha hydroxy acids during the day, which you would apply along with moisturizer and sunscreen each morning. (I will discuss alpha hydroxy acids— mild acids derived from natural substances like fruit, milk, and sugar cane—at length in Chapter 10.) The safety of using tretinoin daily for longer than six months has not really been established. Most dermatologists recommend using tretinoin for six months each year.

Retin-A or Renova costs between $50 and $70 for approximately a six-week supply.

Adjunct Procedures

Because it has been proven to help peeled skin heal faster, tretinoin is frequently used as a pretreatment prior to fruit-acid peels and medium-depth peels. Once the skin has completely healed from any resurfacing or filler procedure, tretinoin is an important part of almost every prescribed maintenance routine.

Frequently Asked Questions about Tretinoin

Are there any side effects or risks?

Being a powerful acid, Retin-A can be expected to produce some degree of redness, flakiness, or irritation, but these problems are not serious and generally subside within a week of treatment.

I have very dark skin. Should I be using tretinoin?
The honest answer is, probably not. You should consult a dermatologist, of course, but so far, unfortunately, Retin-A and Renova have not been carefully studied in people with moderately or darkly pigmented skin. There have been reports that, in some patients, areas treated with tretinoin have developed a temporary increase or decrease in the amount of pigment present. However, the affected areas returned to normal either after tretinoin use was discontinued or after the patient's skin adjusted to the medication.

What are the long-term effects of tretinoin on cell turnover?
Good question. There is a school of thought that believes that, by speeding up cell turnover, tretinoin will actually *advance* the aging process. The logic behind this is that if there is a limited number of times that cells can turn over before they can no longer function, then stimulating cell turnover is not a good idea. However, the few studies of long-term tretinoin use fail to show any negative consequences. This doctor's opinion is that it's well worth the risk.

I have a moisturizer formulated with vitamin A. Is that the same thing as Retin-A?
No. The active ingredient in Retin-A is an acid derived from vitamin A. Vitamin creams—or creams containing retinyl compounds like retinyl acetate—are not proved to do anything for your skin. Save your money or spend it on Retin-A instead.

Should I use an alpha hydroxy acid while using tretinoin?
Again, you might want to consult your dermatologist, but using AHAs in conjunction with tretinoin can be wonderfully effective. A commonly prescribed regimen would have you apply Retin-A nightly for six months and AHA every morning; on the off months, only AHA would be applied once a day, either in the morning or at night. If you have sensitive skin, you might try using Retin-A every other night, with an AHA on the nights between. But AHA or no AHA, remember that using tretinoin must be part of a broad skin-care program that includes regular cleansing, moisturizing, and the religious use of sunscreen.

Is it safe to use tretinoin during pregnancy?
I wouldn't. Safe use of tretinoin during pregnancy has not been demonstrated, and it isn't known whether tretinoin is passed to infants through breast milk.

THE BLEACHES: HQRA CREAM AND OTHER "SPOT" REMOVERS

Freckles may have been cute when you were a kid, but hyperpigmented skin patches on an adult are anything but. What causes age spots (also known as liver spots because of their color, solar lentigines, keratoses, sun spots, and so forth) and other pigment disorders to crop up all over the place as we age? Changes in skin color, also called *chloasma* or *melasma*, result from a host of factors. They assume a number of forms, most of them somewhat unsightly but rarely threatening to your health. Ranging from light brown to black, smooth to rough, unpleasant to horrific, age spots occur primarily as a result of unprotected sun exposure. In women birth-control pills, pregnancy, or estrogen replacement therapy can also lead to an outbreak of brown or ashen patches of skin. They have nothing whatsoever to do with your liver, however.

In most cases age spots occur when the melanocytes in the lower epidermis, fending off the sun's rays, step up their production of melanin, the pigment that gives your skin its color and protects it from ultraviolet exposure. As you may know, the fairer you are, the lighter the concentration of melanin in your skin and the greater your susceptibility to sun damage.

It is not exactly understood what causes melanin production to go awry in the face of excess sun exposure, but when age spots appear, they will not fade on their own, no matter how much sunscreen you cake over them. (*They should, however, serve as a keen reminder of the more serious growths that can develop if you continue to sunbathe unprotected.*) In lighter to olive skin, age spots emerge as relatively small brown growths, flat or raised, that may grow or change shape over time; in darker skin they tend to be ashen gray and blotchy.

Age spots can also appear as areas of hypopigmentation, or pigment loss. More often, though, this condition occurs spontaneously, for reasons that are poorly understood. One such condition, *vitiligo*, is an autoimmune disorder, predominantly afflicting African Americans, that results in patches of sudden—and often total—pigment depletion. Unfortunately restoring skin pigmentation has proved a more intractable problem than decreasing it, but treatments for vitiligo are showing progress.

At Face Value

In mild cases of vitiligo, I usually recommend experimenting with waterproof coverage makeup products, which nowadays exist in a vast range of skin tones and blend astonishingly well into your skin. When vitiligo is severe but covers less than a quarter of the body, dermatologists may try to repigment the affected areas through ultraviolet-A (PUVA) therapy and *psoralens*, a group of chemicals that make the skin sensitive to light. When it covers more than half your body, it may prove easier to lighten the darker areas with a "bleaching" agent like *hydroquinone*, which I will describe in a moment. However, both processes are quite long and involved and should be seriously discussed with your dermatologist.

Similarly *hyperpigmentation* that extends below the epidermis deep into the dermis has proved difficult to lighten or erase. Fortunately, though, age spots are most commonly rooted in the epidermis and are highly treatable. Laser and chemical resurfacing, *curettage* (scraping), and freezing are all effective methods for treating age spots that don't respond to topical treatments (see "Frequently Asked Questions about HQRA" below), but unless the area is severely hyperpigmented, I will always try a bleaching cream first. Bleaching creams that contain hydroquinones plus vitamin A derivative, and vitamin C creams are common weapons in the arsenal against brown spots. I'd like to clarify something. The creams under discussion are really not "bleach." This is a misnomer. When you and I think of bleach, we conjure up an image of a stain on a white shirt where you take the bleach, pour it on, and it removes the stain. This is not doing that. This is not taking out the brown. Rather, it is

(37)

shutting off the manufacturing plant that *makes* the brown, and then the brown has to be sloughed off or shed off over time. That's why if you add Retin-A or exfoliating agents to bleach, the process works a lot faster and a lot better.

Of all the skin-lightening agents, hydroquinone is the most common (kojic acid and azalax acid are also used, but less effectively in my experience) and can be found easily in 1 percent to 2 percent concentration in products at most drugstores under the names Porcelana and Esoterica. In this dosage the agent takes about four weeks to show results. That's because it takes that long for your hyperpigmented cells to shed and new, melanin-inhibited cells to rise to the surface. It is generally safe on all skin colors and types. Your dermatologist may also suggest that you combine a 2 percent hydroquinine lotion with an alpha hydroxy acid or tretinoin to speed up the turnover of discolored cells— a tactic I have found extremely effective. With or without the addition of Retin-A, however, hydroquinone makes the skin highly sensitive to ultraviolet light, which means you should either stay out of the sun or wear sunscreen. Besides, sun exposure only promotes the production of new melanin, which defeats the purpose, wouldn't you say?

If 2 percent hydroquinone combined with tretinoin or an AHA doesn't cut it—and even if your age spots aren't that severe, it might well not—you may need a prescription-strength (3 percent to 4 percent) hydroquinone formula to get the job done. In my office I generally prescribe HQRA cream, a combination of 4 percent hydroquinone cream, .05 percent Retin-A cream, and 2½ percent hydrocortisone cream that has proved superbly effective in fading or eliminating keratoses, some kinds of birthmarks, hormonal discolorations, and even darkened scars. The hydrocortisone in the compound, which some of you hemorrhoid sufferers will recognize, is a powerful soothing agent that will prevent the formula from irritating or overdrying the skin, which may occur to some extent at the beginning of HQRA treatment. Meanwhile, the Retin-A exfoliates the discolored areas and works to restore the texture of the de-spotted skin surface. A winning combination.

HQRA cream is a safe but powerful drug. Any dermatologist prescribing it should give you specific instructions regarding how many times a day to use the cream, over what periods of time, and on which particular areas of your body. Not all age spots will require hydroquinone in this dosage, after all, and there is no sense in using it on areas where a less expensive, over-the-counter concentration of hydroquinone will do the trick.

Directions for Using Bleach

Generally HQRA is applied once a day, before bedtime, on clean, dry skin. Before you begin your HQRA treatment, the product should be skin-tested by spreading a thin film of the cream on your forearm before bedtime each night for three consecutive nights. If you notice mild itching and redness, you have nothing to worry about. If, however, you notice moderate to severe redness, swelling, itching, or hives, you should consult your dermatologist before proceeding with treatment. As with tretinoin, before applying HQRA you'll need to wash your face with a gentle cleanser or mild soap and pat it dry. Then, you simply apply a thin film with your fingertip to each affected area. Be extremely careful to avoid getting the cream in your eyes or the corners of your mouth. You may want to apply the cream every other night until you feel that your skin tolerates the chemical and that it can be safely applied nightly.

Because HQRA is a potent bleaching and exfoliating agent, it is more essential than ever to use an SPF 15 sunscreen during treatment. Otherwise, your skin will be even more susceptible to sunburn and subsequent sun damage and discoloration. HQRA should produce visible results within four weeks, but—fair warning—it may take many months before your dark spots have lightened acceptably or disappeared.

HQRA costs $100 for a two-month supply.

Related Procedures

Hydroquinone treatments can be safely combined with exfoliants like Retin-A and alpha hydroxy acids and the whole range of "filler" techniques. HQRA therapy combined with a light chemical peel is a potent combination for reversing early but marked sun damage. Tretinoin therapy combined with a deeper chemical peel may be preferred over hydroquinone therapy when significant spotting is accompanied by an abundance of wrinkles.

Frequently Asked Questions about HQRA

Are there any side effects or risks?

Studies of the long-term safety of hydroquinone use are still ongoing but so far have failed to turn up any cause for alarm. In rare cases long-term hydroquinone use has, strangely enough, caused the skin to darken. If you're using an over-the-counter product and you see no improvement after two months, I would consult a dermatologist. With a prescription treatment like HQRA, your dermatologist should be monitoring your progress anyway.

Are there any age spot compounds made especially for women with dark or black skin?
In fact, there are. I will refrain from naming brands here, but there are quite a few skin-lightening products out there, many using hydroquinone, that have been developed for black skin. Look for one in an emollient base that also contains an alpha hydroxy acid and an anti-inflammatory like hydrocortisone; the combination has proved quite effective on darker skin tones. If over-the-counter hydroquinone products don't do the trick, however, you probably shouldn't up the dosage. Studies have shown that hydroquinone in concentrations above 3 percent may actually worsen discolorations in dark-skinned women. In any event, at that point you'll need to consult a dermatologist.

What shouldn't I do while I'm using hydroquinone?
Aside from discontinuing unprotected sun exposure, you must not use abrasive cleansers on any discolored area. *Do not use any hydroquinone product at all if you are pregnant, trying to become pregnant, or nursing.*

If hydroquinone doesn't work, what should I try next?
Don't fret. You still have plenty of options, albeit more costly. On particularly rough or intractable growths, your dermatologist may opt to pretreat the spotted area with Retin-A for two to four weeks, followed by a salicylic acid or

trichloroacetic (TCA) *acid peel* or some combination thereof. This procedure causes the spots to blister before they fade, which can be painful, but it works very well. Or your dermatologist may recommend a course of *laser treatment* (which we will describe later in the chapter), a more expensive but virtually painless procedure that zaps hyperpigmented cells into oblivion. The number of laser sessions required is contingent upon the depth and severity of your discoloration, but it tends to carry the smallest risk of scarring. However, it is not recommended when spots are bumpy or raised. Finally, there's *liquid nitrogen.* Some dermatologists consider "freezing" age spots an outmoded procedure, but it does work better on some types of growths. Not surprisingly it carries the risk of destroying too much melanin and leaving the treated area with a white, frostbitten look.

THE POWER OF (CHEMICAL) PEELING

Although a new breed of laser treatments is gradually taking the place of this decades-old wrinkle remedy, chemical peeling remains an incredibly effective and widely used technique for improving or erasing wrinkles and age spots. Known also as *chemical facial rejuvenation, chemabrasion,* and somewhat inaccurately, as *"chemosurgery,"* this extraordinary process relies on the penetration of an irritating exfoliant into the skin, producing a controlled wound that brings about a generalized tissue regeneration. The result: smoother, revitalized skin.

The chemical peel has its roots in antiquity. The ancient Egyptians used animal oils, salt, and alabaster to rejuvenate the skin. Ancient Egyptian women bathed in sour milk, unknowingly making use of one of today's most widely used alpha hydroxy acids (lactic). Turks used fire to singe the skin in their painful-sounding version of exfoliation. And ancient Greek noblewomen experimented with overnight masks of many sorts, one of which consisted of a bedtime facial that was scrubbed off the following morning with asses' milk!

Chemical peeling, as we know it, however, began with the discovery of *phenol* in Germany at the turn of the twentieth century, when aesthetic surgery and dermatology were just assuming their modern form. During World War I, phenol solutions were used to treat gunpowder burns to the face. By the late 1930s the chemical peel was already laying waste to wrinkles in salons all over Europe and the United States. In the ensuing years dermatologists refined the treatment exponentially, developing an entire range of exfoliating agents and therapies.

These days we can choose, with great precision, how deep we want a peel to go. There are *three basic types of peels— light, medium,* and *deep*—and the depth of your peel depends on the extent of your wrinkling and sun damage. However, not all light, medium, or deep peels are performed in the same manner; within each type the course of treatment and concentration of the chemical agent can vary to a degree. Still, the intended effect for each kind of peel is predictable and precise. *Light peels*—which use different combinations of low-strength chemical agents like trichloroacetic acid (TCA), salicylic acid, alpha hydroxy acids, and resorcinol— target the stratum corneum, the top layer of packed dead skin cells, to restore the skin's luster and remove superficial lines and discolorations; in some cases they can also incidentally improve the collagen below the epidermis. *Medium-depth peels* generally use TCA, sometimes combined with phenol, to penetrate to the lower papillary layer and upper dermis, eliminating deeper wrinkles and discolorations and enhancing overall skin elasticity. Finally, *deep peels*, which are best suited to very fair, thin-skinned women, penetrate to the deep reticular dermis, essentially dissolving the epidermis along the way; in addition to rejuvenating the stratum corneum, the healing process that follows increases and rearranges the collagen below, thus improving the skin's tautness as well as tone.

There are, of course, risks involved in all of these procedures, and you should familiarize yourself with them before opting to undergo even a superficial peel. In fact, of all the treatments discussed in this book, medium and deep peels carry the highest risk of complications and, for all intents and purposes, should be considered surgical. Among dark-skinned patients in particular, the deeper the peel, the higher the risk of losing skin color—sometimes for good. Still, provided that your doctor regularly performs these procedures, is sensitive to your skin color and type, and knows every aspect of your medical history, all should go smoothly.

LIGHT PEELS

Before I describe this terrific procedure, I want to clear up one point of confusion. Although the two are easily confused because of some overlap in chemicals and methodology, a light chemical peel is not the same thing as an alpha hydroxy acid peel, which I consider a preventive treatment and will discuss later on in Chapter 10, "Inventions and Pre-ventions." Put briefly, the AHA peel (performed often with glycolic acid) is a cosmetic rather than medical procedure now performed at salons just about everywhere, and while it does temporarily improve the skin's texture and tone by encouraging cell turnover, it doesn't really "peel" the super-ficial or light skin at all. This is not to say that AHA peels are ineffective or frivolous, but for all that money spent, you'll see few really dramatic results. After all, if they pene-trated any deeper than the skin's outmost exterior, they would be classified as drugs and regulated by the FDA. As of now, they're not.

All of which is to say that the only person who should per-form an actual peel on your skin is a medical doctor. No exceptions. I'm not knocking salons, which can be very relax-ing and make your skin look great, but there is increasing concern among dermatologists and plastic surgeons about salons that are performing high-strength peels better left to qualified doctors. There is even some feeling that salon peels, no matter what strength, should be banned altogether.

That said, the medically performed light chemical peel is still reasonably light. It removes only the stratum cor-neum (the dead outer layer of the epidermis), sending a mes-sage down to the basal-layer cells (the growing, living layer of the epidermis) to stimulate their metabolic rate. This creates younger, fresher-looking skin, producing a result equivalent to using Retin-A for one year. It leaves the skin lustrous and glowing, lightening, and in some cases remov-ing, superficial lentigines ("sun spots"), hyperpigmentations, blemishes, and very fine lines. Skin tone becomes more even and its texture smoother. However, the light chemical peel will not remove deep wrinkles or scars, since they reside within the dermis.

The light chemical peel can be performed on all skin types and colors, without exception. In darker-skinned patients, light peels may cause minimal, but often only temporary, dyspigmentations; deeper peels pose a much greater risk, often causing severe losses of color in black or Hispanic patients. All peels are absolutely contraindicated for pregnant or nursing women; and if you suffer from eczema or psoriasis, or if you are allergic to aspirin, appropriate precautions should be taken. The typical procedure takes one visit, lasts thirty to forty-five minutes, and is done in the doctor's office. If your sun damage is very minimal, your dermatologist might recommend a biweekly series of lighter peels instead, followed by a course of tretinoin and alpha hydroxy acids to enhance and maintain the effects. In most cases, though, this is a one-shot peel.

The Procedure

For two weeks prior to the procedure, you will be instructed to apply Retin-A cream (.05 percent) twice a day to ensure a more even peel, and you'll be given a prescription for Zovirax to prevent a herpes simplex infection. Right before the procedure, the skin is cleansed with soap and water to remove any dirt and makeup, followed by a cleansing with acetone to remove excess lipids and sebum. The light chemical peel agent (in my practice a combination of fruit acids and diluted tricholoracetic acid) is then applied with a cotton-tipped applicator or gauze. There will be a slight burning sensation, lasting only five to ten minutes; a fan is used during the procedure (and compresses and creams are applied afterward) to cool the skin. Initially the skin will appear frosty white, but within fifteen minutes it will turn rosy red. In the next two to three days, it will become a tan to darkish brown. By the third day, peeling will begin around the eyes, nose, and mouth. From then on, the skin will peel off in sheets, like a shedding snake's. Not very pretty perhaps, but not as bad as it sounds by any stretch.

Within seven to ten days, the peeling process will be completed, and the skin will have a pink appearance. Since the peeling doesn't begin until the third day after the procedure, if you have it done on a Wednesday, you could go to work that day and on Thursday and Friday. But bear in mind that your skin will look tan, dry, and tight. Each day it will get progressively flakier, although most of the major peeling will occur over the weekend. Provided that you avoid sun exposure, there will be no medical reason to stay indoors, but only you can decide how comfortable you feel about "appearing in public" during the peeling process. During the peeling period, you cannot wear cosmetics and must rinse your face very gently. After the peeling is complete, your skin will look brighter, and most brown marks will be gone. Your new skin will still be extrasensitive to the sun, though, so it will be vital to wear an SPF 15 sunscreen outdoors (reapplied every two hours), and don't forget your sun hat. Do not schedule your peel closer than six weeks before a planned sun-filled vacation.

The procedure generally costs between $400 and $800.

Related Procedures

The light chemical peel is often effectively enhanced through selective laser resurfacing (to wipe out stubborn crow's-feet); fat, collagen, or Botox injections (to fill out those areas of the face that have markedly lost fat); and vitamin injections (see the section on *mesotherapy* later in the chapter) to regenerate collagen and elastin and thus slow down the development of future wrinkles. Tretinoin therapy (bleaching) will also help maintain the benefits of any peel, once the skin is fully healed.

Frequently Asked Questions about the Light Chemical Peel
Are there any side effects or risks?
Possible side effects are hyperpigmentations (which may be bleached) and broken capillaries (which may be treated with electrodesiccation). There is a slight risk of herpes infections (which may be prevented with Zovirax capsules) and bacterial infections (which may be prevented with prophylactic antibiotics).

How long do the results last?
A light chemical peel should be repeated every twelve months in most people between the ages of thirty and fifty. After fifty optimal results last about six months, when the procedure may be repeated. Results improve with each repetition.

Do I have to peel my entire face, or can I peel just one area?
It is possible to peel a particular region of the face, but usually, to minimize the risk of uneven coloration and ensure "cosmetic blending," I recommend peeling the entire face at once.

Can I have a light peel while I am pregnant or nursing?
Absolutely not.

Is the light peel covered by insurance?
No. All chemical peels are considered cosmetic procedures.

Where else on the body can it be done?
In addition to the face, the neck, hands, chest, elbows, knees, back, and arms can be effectively treated in this way.

THE MEDIUM-DEPTH PEEL

In terms of technique and healing process, the medium-depth peel varies very little from the light peel. The most significant difference between them is that the medium peel, like the deep peel, is not recommended for people with olive-to-dark skin. As with the light peel, the skin is preoperatively prepped with Retin-A for two to three weeks in order to enhance the skin's response to and recovery from the procedure. However, since the chemical agent used here, usually some combination of TCA and phenol, is designed to penetrate the upper portion of the dermis to improve or eliminate deeper lines and folds, the medium-depth peel is unquestionably more painful and involved. The addition of phenol to the equation also brings with it a host of possible complications—the risk of depigmentation, for example—that must be taken into account.

Whereas the light peel is performed in less than forty-five minutes, using only a fan to cool the treated area, the medium-depth peel takes about an hour and a half and usually requires some sort of anesthesia, usually in the form of "nerve blocks" or intravenous sedation. Many practitioners are able to reduce anxiety and pain merely through diazepam or aspirin, or even by talking to their patients during the procedure, but the point is that some discomfort is inevitable. Furthermore, while both light and medium peels carry a similar postpeel recovery period of seven to ten days, redness can persist for up to sixteen weeks with the medium peel (compared to six days with the light peel). On the other hand, the results of the medium-depth peel, often very dramatic, can last from five to ten years. With the light peel you're looking at a year and a half, tops, before you'll want to do it all over again.

My feeling, though, is that if a medium peel is right for you, and you're willing to endure the discomfort, you might as well opt for a deep peel, which affords much better and longer-lasting results. The risks and costs are comparable and the recovery times roughly the same.

The medium-depth peel costs anywhere between $3,500 and $5,000.

THE DEEP PEEL

The deep peel is a potent and controversial procedure that has fallen into considerable disfavor over the years. Some of the vehement criticism launched against it has been valid, some of it simple hysteria. By now, though, the complications associated with deep peels are widely known, and no good dermatologist will downplay them. The root of the problem is that phenol, the powerful agent invariably used in deep peels to undo profound wrinkles and even tighten loose skin, is a *melanocyte* destroyer, which can cause significant loss of pigmentation in the treated area. Naturally this makes it inadvisable to treat only part of the face. But even performing a full-face phenol peel can mean a color contrast at the jawline. Further complicating matters, the phenol-treated area is routinely covered with a nonporous tape to enhance the chemical's effectiveness, rendering it even more difficult to monitor and control the depth of penetration. To top it all off, if applied too suddenly, phenol can cause a cardiac arrhythmia.

It's no picnic, I realize. Notwithstanding these risks, however, deep peels really do work, and work remarkably well. The procedure is still not recommended for people with olive or dark skin, but if your complexion is fair, your eyes light, and your wrinkles severe, you're an ideal candidate. The list of complications associated with deep peeling has become far less menacing over the past decade, as dermatologists have developed phenol preparations whose effects are less caustic and easier to manage.

Phenol has been around for more than ninety years now, and the fact that it's still around, and still widely used in various formulations, speaks volumes. In my office I have had great success with Baker's formula, a popular combination designed specifically for deep peels. Baker's formula consists of phenol, water, croton oil, and septisol. Cautiously applied and monitored, it essentially dissolves the epidermis and upper third of the dermis, which are then regenerated from the lining of the hair follicles deep within the dermis. During the procedure, which takes two to three hours because the phenol must be applied gradually, your heart will be closely monitored for reaction to the toxicity, but the risk of arrhythmia is slight. With the help of local and intravenous anesthesia, you won't feel or remember a thing. As the skin heals, new collagen bands are produced, making the new dermis thicker and more elastic, and the stratum corneum above it grows back tighter and smoother. Superficial and medium-depth wrinkles are removed, and deep folds are significantly softened. In short, it works.

I should say right here that more and more dermatologists now prefer lasers to deep peeling to correct severe sun damage and wrinkling, because they offer more predictable results and easier healing. However, deep peeling is still widely requested and performed and remains an excellent option for wrinkle-ridden skin.

The best candidate for a deep chemical peel is a fair-complexioned, light-eyed, thin-skinned person. Does this mean that if your skin is olive- or dark-hued, the procedure's absolutely off-limits? Naturally that's a determination a dermatologist must make on a case-by-case basis, but the answer is, don't get your hopes up. Although the lines may improve to an excellent degree, a deep peel done on dark skin carries a considerable risk of dispigmentation.

Contraindications

If you have a heart, liver, or kidney condition or are pregnant, phenol peels should be avoided altogether. Before you undergo any peeling procedure, your doctor should grill you on your medical history, asking specifically whether you have any health problems that may interfere with your convalescence and/or necessitate a consultation with an internist prior to treatment. Your doctor should also ask you whether you are allergic to any medications and describe each phase of the procedure in detail, from preoperative analgesia through the (at times uncomfortable) healing period. Finally, he or she should note your expectations and be clear with you about which aging signs the procedure will and will not reverse.

The Procedure

As with the light peel, you will be instructed to use Retin-A twice a day for two weeks before the procedure and to take Zovirax. The deep peel takes two to three hours and is generally done in the doctor's office. Right before the procedure, you will be given a mild intravenous sedative and local "nerve block"; anesthesia will be administered to your entire face. After the skin is thoroughly cleansed with acetone, the phenol peel begins. The Baker's formula is applied in sections, at fifteen-minute intervals, until the entire face is peeled; all the while an anesthesiologist should be monitoring your blood pressure and pulse.

Once the peel is complete, an occlusive waterproof tape may be gently applied to the face in wide strips. This optional mask, which is left in place for forty-eight hours, enhances the peel's penetration. After it is removed, you will apply an antibacterial powder mask for the next three days (you'll also take an oral antibiotic), until your skin is fully crusted over. During this period it is important to keep your head elevated during sleep. On the fifth day, warm compresses are applied to the face three times a day, and you will begin moisturizing with that most trusted of emollients, Crisco.

Fair warning: your face will look greatly swollen and ugly for a little while, but within twelve days the crust sloughs off and the skin is healed and has a bright red and smooth appearance. That redness usually lasts about a month and may even persist for up to four months, but it is easily concealed with makeup. Then again, you'll look so much (in most cases between ten and fifteen years) younger that some lingering irritation may not bother you at all.

In all, the deep peel will put you out of commission for about two weeks. As with other peels, your new skin will be exquisitely sensitive to the sun, requiring an SPF 15 sunscreen and, preferably, a sun hat whenever you are outdoors. When the skin is fully healed, you'll also want to begin using AHAs and tretinoin to keep the skin exfoliating and healthy.

The deep chemical peel generally costs between $3,500 and $7,500.

Related Procedures

A deep chemical facial peel should be powerful enough to eliminate the need for any complementary facial-resurfacing procedures. However, while radically improving the skin's texture and tone, it may not be able to fully repair sagging skin. Once the skin is healed, a minor face-lift can help tighten whatever loose skin the phenol peel failed to improve.

Frequently Asked Questions about the Deep Chemical Peel

Are there any side effects or risks?

The possible side effects of deep peeling are cardiac arrhythmias, pigmentary alteration, hypertrophic scarring, milia (little white cysts caused by a blockage of hair follicles or sweat glands), herpes simplex and bacterial infections, and prolonged redness and sun sensitivity. All are extremely manageable with careful monitoring, appropriate wound care, and antibiotics.

Is deep peeling painful?
It sounds infinitely more painful than it is. The procedure itself, performed under intravenous sedation and local anesthetic, is virtually painless. After the procedure a mild pain pill is generally needed for twenty-four hours. As I said, your skin will look fairly hideous for a few days—a fact that will cause you more emotional than physical discomfort—but it'll be over before you know it.

Why should I have a deep peel done instead of a face-lift?
Face-lift surgery also produces excellent results, but keep in mind that it will not make your skin itself look any younger. A face-lift is designed to tighten loose skin, and at that it may work wonders, but it will not improve the skin's essential thickness, elasticity, or texture. What's more, face-lifting procedures will do little for fine wrinkles and only minimally improve the nasolabial fold. By contrast, chemical peels, which work by inducing the skin to heal itself, bring about marked improvements above and below the skin surface. They're also significantly less costly than facial surgery.

How long do the results last?
The effects of a deep chemical peel generally last about ten years, at which time they can be safely performed again.

Who should perform my deep peel?
Ah, a good question with a simple answer: a plastic surgeon or dermatologist who has been trained in the art of

chemical peeling, and no one else. Steer clear of salons promising "deep peels." And don't be bashful about asking your dermatologist how regularly he or she performs the procedure.

Do not forget that this is a serious procedure with serious risks.

Mechanical Resurfacing

Again, the object of mechanical resurfacing, which includes dermabrasion and the use of lasers, is similar to the chemical peel: to exfoliate (remove) the top layer or layers of skin, allowing fresh new skin to appear at the surface and the underlying collagen to respond by increasing in area, to bring better tone to the structure beneath the skin. This controlled wounding of the skin heals with cosmetic improvement.

MICRODERMABRASION

Microdermabrasion (also known as "power peeling") exfoliates the skin using crushed crystals of either aluminum oxide or sodium bicarbonate. The procedure is done using a small instrument, almost like a tiny Dust Buster, which is turned on and passed over the face, back and forth. Inside the machine are little crystals, which in a sense sandblast the outer skin, removing it. The machine then basically sucks up the dull, dead skin along with the little crystals. The depth of the dermabrasion depends on the strength to which you set the crystals. In other words, you can set the machine on gentle sandblasting or deep sandblasting, and the results will vary accordingly. Most aestheticians who do this procedure set the strength on very gentle sandblasting because they don't want the client to be uncomfortable or irritated. But that means only a very superficial layer of skin is taken off. One of the problems I have with the procedure as performed in salons is that you can't always see what you're doing, which means less control for the operator.

Still, it's very popular because the machines are inexpensive to buy, and the staff can operate them. So it's something new on the block, which, for my money, is no better than chemical peels and not as good as laser facials.

DERMABRASION: TO SAND OR NOT TO SAND?

Dermabrasion is for deeper scars and deeper wrinkles, severe sun damage, precancerous growths, and uneven skin color. Some call it time-honored, some call it outmoded. With the development of laser treatments, collagen, and lighter-depth peels, most dermatologists, myself included, have hung up their wire brushes for good. A small contingent, however, still swears by dermabrasion as the best remedy for the spot treatment of deep wrinkles. Introduced in 1953, dermabrasion was, for a good while, the only technique other than phenol that effectively rubbed out wrinkles, and it worked quite well. Of course, advances in equipment design and wound care have vastly improved the treatment over the past five decades, but the idea is much the same.

Think of dermabrasion as a high-powered mechanical exfoliating scrub. Like a deep or medium-depth peel, the procedure can improve skin texture and tone, eliminate or soften wrinkles and expression lines, and eradicate age spots. The technique involves no more than using a motorized, handheld rotating metal brush to "sand" the skin. That may sound like some kind of Gothic torture technique, but because no chemicals are involved, dermabrasion is actually safer in some ways than the phenol peel. However, the long-term benefits of dermabrasion don't seem to be on a par with those of phenol peels, which do a much better job of helping the skin generate and lay down new bands of collagen. In any event, both phenol and dermabrasion are becoming equally rarefied as lasers continue to revolutionize the field of *cutaneous resurfacing*.

One area in which dermabrasion has served a particularly useful role is in treating scars, acne scars especially, and expression lines around the mouth. However, deep-pitted scars may require some preliminary treatment, such as "punch" elevation or replacement grafts, before being *dermabraded*. And the fact is that wrinkles, isolated or otherwise, respond so much more reliably to the new breed of lasers that dermabrasion, though indeed effective, is a second-rate option.

The dermabrasion procedure is very simple and most often performed under local anesthesia. Many doctors administer intravenous sedation or general anesthesia before the procedure, however. The dermatologist then "prechills" the skin with ice packs or crushed ice for thirty minutes to enhance the effect of a subsequent refrigerant spray that both anesthetizes and hardens the surface to be dermabraded. Alternatively the doctor may administer nerve blocks to numb the treated area, along with a *tumescent anesthesia*, which also firms up the skin surface. Then the buzzing gets under way.

Using a wire brush or a tool called a diamond fraise, the doctor dermabrades the skin up to, but not beyond, the *midreticular dermis.* Once the dermabrasion is complete, the face will look an utter mess, but it is quickly wrapped in a soothing dressing (called *Vigilon*), which usually eliminates the need for pain medication. The next day the dressing is removed, a petrolatum ointment is applied, and the face is covered with a clean cotton mask. The patient will then follow an at-home regimen of cleansing the area and reapplying the ointment at intervals to keep the skin from forming a crust. Within eight days the dermabraded skin heals but will look red for a good few months. Normal activity can be resumed, but unprotected sun exposure is again a no-no.

Related Procedures

Like chemical peels of all depths, dermabrasion can be enhanced through face-lifting procedures to correct sagging skin. Filler techniques of all sorts, vitamin injections, and tretinoin all are helpful as well. Patients with a tendency toward hyperpigmentation or *melasma* are generally started on hydroquinone as soon as the skin is healed.

Frequently Asked Questions about Dermabrasion

Are there any side effects or risks?

Frequent postoperative conditions include intense redness, which usually disappears within two months, and *milial* cysts—little collections of dead skin that occlude the pore. (The cysts are usually rapidly responsive to tretinoin.) There is also a risk of herpes simplex, which can be prevented entirely through preoperative antiviral drugs. As with the medium-depth or deep chemical peel, there is also a significant risk of pigment alteration. That is why this procedure is best suited to fair skin and best performed over the entire face. If you're dark-skinned, some mild version of dermabrasion can be safely done, but the risk of depigmentation is still high enough to make the procedure ill-advised. Finally, there is a small risk of hypertrophic scarring, almost always correctable through topical corticosteroids or laser treatment.

I've heard that dermabrasion is good for isolated groups of wrinkles—"whistle lines," for instance. Is that true?

Well, it is and it isn't. It is true that many doctors successfully use dermabrasion to eliminate wrinkles around the mouth, finding the technique easier to manage than the chemical peels for spot treatments. Similarly dermabrasion has proved more effective than peeling for smoothing acne scars. However, as with the deeper peels, the risk of pigment alteration is high, which makes it risky to dermabrade only part of the face. And if you're going to resurface your whole face, you're far better off doing it with a laser.

Laser Resurfacing

HOW LASERS WORK

I realize it's been a while since you dozed off in high school physics, so I'll refresh your memory. A *laser*, which stands for *l*ight *a*mplification by *s*timulated *e*mission of *r*adiation, is a device that harnesses electromagnetic radiation of mixed frequencies into a highly amplified, integrated beam. First formulated in Einstein's famous 1916 paper on quantum theory, lasers were invented to produce specific wavelengths of light at specific energy levels, each with its own function or application. The first practical uses of lasers in the early 1960s were in medicine, when ophthalmologists successfully employed them in the treatment of retinal blood vessel problems of diabetics. Nowadays, of course, lasers are ubiquitous, used in everything from high-tech weaponry to bar code scanners at the supermarket checkout. In nearly every medical discipline, they have become an invaluable tool for carefully dividing or welding tissues or destroying specific tissue cells.

No longer considered a new technique, laser resurfacing of the skin has recently surpassed chemical peels as the most sought-after nonsurgical method of rejuvenation. In the year 2001, U.S. dermatologists and plastic surgeons performed some one hundred thousand laser peels, and the procedure is only getting hotter. And with good reason. Easily customized and controlled, the nonspreading, visible light of a computer-controlled laser beam affords the doctor the unprecedented ability to take aim at wrinkles while leaving healthy surrounding tissues unscathed. Remember that the biggest problem with the chemical peel arsenal is control and healing time—that different skin types react differently to the peeling process, which in itself is difficult to fine-tune. With lasers, by contrast, a well-trained physician can successfully vaporize or ablate exceedingly thin layers of skin at a time, allowing the depth of penetration to be precisely controlled. This means better results with far less discomfort and a far speedier recovery.

Lasers of varying strengths have been employed in cosmetic procedures for more than twenty years now. Not all of these generate an emission truly gentle enough for the skin. Until very recently, the most trusted and popular laser for resurfacing and wrinkle removal was the carbon dioxide (CO_2) laser, which was developed with *cutaneous* resurfacing specifically in mind. The initial round of CO_2 lasers, known as *continuous wave lasers*, still caused considerable thermal damage, and their use was restricted to the removal of non-facial birthmarks, port-wine stains (caused by enlarged blood vessels), and tattoos. But within a few years, the advent of pulsed and superpulsed CO_2 lasers, which deliver a rapid, computer-generated pattern of energy that mini-mizes tissue burning, changed all that. Suddenly plastic sur-geons and dermatologists had an incredible, FDA-approved tool for aggressively and accurately treating the entire gamut of aging symptoms, from sun spots to deep creases, lip lines to eyelid folds. What's more, the CO_2 laser could be safely passed over extensive regions of skin, even the entire face. This distinguished it from previous lasers designed to zap only isolated flaws. Before long the CO_2 laser's high-intensity beams outsizzled its chemical counterparts, emerg-ing for a time as the be-all and end-all of wrinkle removers.

That is, until the *erbium YAG laser* came along. Although still widely used today for spot treatments as well as full-facial resurfacing—and with excellent results, at that—the CO_2 laser is now on the way out. The new kid on the block, the erbium YAG laser, which arrived in 1996, is probably the best weapon in the knifeless fight for fresher, younger-looking skin. Named for its components—erbium, yttrium, aluminum, and garnet—the erbium YAG laser deploys a beam that can be adjusted, as never before, to selectively penetrate the skin with varying degrees of heat. Like the CO_2 laser, the erbium YAG laser works by emitting short bursts of high-energy light that vaporize skin cells. But where the CO_2 laser was precise, the erbium laser is exacting, affording a degree of control that makes its predecessors look sloppy. With better results than chemical or fruit-acid peels, at a fraction of the discomfort, this remarkable device can be set to penetrate only as deeply as needed, and it can also be individualized for each person's skin tone, sensitivity, or specific problems. It also makes it possible to "scan" and target specific creases and discolorations as the procedure is being performed. For age spots and uneven skin tones, lines and wrinkles, acne scarring, spider veins, and port-wine stains—you name the symptom, and the erbium laser will beam it away, leaving your skin noticeably tighter, smoother, and fresher-looking.

As you can tell, I'm a big fan of this laser.

Why is the erbium YAG laser so much better? Without getting too technical, I'll try to explain. The water in your skin cells—which are mostly water—absorbs laser light. But the heat generated by CO_2 lasers is not effectively absorbed, and a large amount of its energy can affect the surrounding tissue, leading to painful thermal damage that increases healing time and decreases the procedure's effectiveness. As I have noted, the CO_2 laser is, relatively speaking, a minimally painful technique that produces excellent results. But the erbium YAG laser, which generates the exact wavelength of light optimally absorbed by water, directs and distributes its energy with incomparable consistency and selectivity. As a result, it can penetrate the skin only thirty-millionths of an inch at a time and scatter next to no damaging heat in the process. In other words, it can seek and destroy wrinkles of any depth without the extensive incidental burning caused by a TCA peel or even the CO_2 laser.

Of course, even with the erbium YAG laser, not every result is a miracle, and the chance of scarring or permanent pigmentary changes persists, but no device available to cosmetic dermatology has reduced these risks more substantially. Simply put, there is no other laser in its class.

The Procedure

The erbium YAG laser procedure is straightforward and can be performed in a doctor's office. Depending on the purpose for which it is being performed, the procedure can take anywhere from a few minutes for a minor problem to an hour or so for more extensive treatment.

I use a local or topical anesthetic to numb the skin and, if necessary, a mild sedative. Discomfort is minor during and after the procedure, but if treatment is extensive, an anesthetist may be used. The level of discomfort varies from person to person and depends largely on what area is being treated, but most patients forgo pain medication entirely during this procedure, comparing the discomfort to a sunburn or mild rash. A good number of patients, however, opt for a local anesthetic or topical numbing agent. Once programmed, the computerized laser is then coursed over the entire surface being treated, usually with repeated passes over stubborn spots and deep wrinkles. The length of the procedure is proportional to the size of the area being treated, but for a full-face zap, it takes about an hour. After the procedure, the skin will appear pink, but just how pink, raw, swollen, or crusty depends on the depth of the treatment.

One thing to keep in mind: with lasers it is critically

important to find a doctor who's using lasers every day. I can't stress this advice enough. Although no certification is required to perform laser procedures—all you need is a medical license and the cost of the machine—the learning curve with lasers is unmistakably steep, and results are directly proportional to the doctor's facility with the device. So don't be afraid to put a prospective doctor through the mill, asking pointed questions about his or her training and specific experience with the laser. Again, the beauty of the laser is that you can tell it exactly what to do if you know how. In my practice, where it has rapidly become a mainstay, I use the erbium YAG in an entire line of treatments, from the much-publicized laser facial, a terrific ten-minute procedure that vaporizes only the stratum corneum, to deep full-face resurfacing, from acne treatments to spot and scar removal. Whether it's vaporizing wrinkles, lentigines, or clogged pores, it removes defects with unparalleled selectivity. To be sure, as with any medical procedure, you should discuss any questions or concerns you have about the erbium YAG laser with your physician, but if he or she has enjoyed using this high-tech tool as much as I have, you will quickly be put at ease.

Erbium YAG laser treatment remains quite costly, as the machines cost about $100,000 apiece. At $200 a quick laser facial is very reasonable, but a full-face resurfacing may run you $2,500—three or four times the cost of a TCA peel. Still, it's considerably cheaper than a face-lift, and with proper skin care, the results of laser resurfacing can be good for up to ten years. Factor in the quicker healing time and relatively pain-free procedure, and the laser's tough to resist.

Related Procedures

The erbium YAG laser can be used in conjunction with almost any surgical or nonsurgical cosmetic procedure, from Botox injections to face-lifts. However, in the right doctor's hands, the erbium YAG laser is so accurate, effective, and versatile that, depending on the extent of your skin damage, it may eliminate the need for any additional therapies.

Frequently Asked Questions about Erbium YAG Lasers

Will there be any pain postoperatively?

Not generally.

When will I see results? How long will they last?

Noticeable results are seen within a few days, and even with the deepest erbium peels, you can expect to be completely healed within a few weeks. Light resurfacing around the eyes and lips, a commonly performed procedure with this laser, takes only a few days to heal, meaning you can have the procedure done on a Friday morning and expect to be in good shape by Monday morning.

In any case, after laser treatment you'll still need to be very careful to protect your new skin, avoiding sun exposure as much as possible and wearing doctor-recommended sunscreens whenever you are outside. Remember that sun damage was the reason you had the procedure done in the first place!

Are there any side effects or risks?

With the CO_2 laser, there was a small but notable risk of transient hyperpigmentation, or spotting, which could usually be treated with hydroquinone or some other bleaching agent. There was also a risk of scarring, burns, and in rare cases, the paralysis of certain facial nerves. Although similar complications can occur with the erbium YAG laser, it has substantially diminished the risks of laser resurfacing. Again, as with CO_2 lasers, *it is positively vital to find a physician who's using the erbium YAG laser every day,* as there is a significant learning curve with the procedure. And with the deeper erbium YAG laser peels, it is crucially important to adhere closely to your doctor's postoperative regimen, to avert delayed healing, infection, or scarring.

I've heard that laser resurfacing is the only nonsurgical option for sagging skin. Is that true?

It is true. But with a caveat. I'm the first to admit that, for seriously loose skin, there is not a lot the dermatological arsenal—even the laser—can do. As I've said, from time to time I'll recommend that a patient undergo a chemical or light laser peel to rejuvenate her skin and then ship her off to a plastic surgeon to tighten her jawline, neck, cheeks, or brow. Unlike previous lasers, however, the erbium YAG has also shown a lot of promise in the sagging skin department. For reasons not entirely understood, the intense heat generated by lasers tautens the skin and stimulates collagen production more effectively than chemical peels. Although for extreme wrinkling or sagging, as seen in turkey neck, a facelift is still the better option, it is well worth investigating whether the erbium YAG laser can iron out your loose skin.

What is this "laser facial" I've heard so much about?
The laser facial has my patients hooked, and with good reason. The extremely precise erbium YAG laser is capable of vaporizing the outer-outermost layer of the epidermis. In doing just that (with the help of a mild heat-conducting skin preparation), this ten-minute procedure, safe enough to be repeated every six weeks, keeps the skin miraculously soft and smooth. After the laser facial, the skin will be pinkish for roughly twenty-four hours, but side effects are exceedingly rare. Far more effective than the fruit-acid facials performed at most salons, the laser facial effectively exfoliates the skin, dissolving blackheads and whiteheads along the way.

I have dark skin. Can I be treated with the erbium YAG laser?
Yes. With previous lasers deeper-pigmented skin types regularly suffered pigmentation irregularities following laser resurfacing. In black skin in particular, lasers such as the CO_2, due to the intense heat of their beams, were associated with the formation of hard, raised scars called keloids. So they were recommended only to men and women with fair, nonoily skin. By contrast, the erbium YAG laser, which can be fine-tuned for each individual's skin tone, has proved extremely safe on very dark skin of varying types. If you have olive or black skin, it is all the more important to find a skilled laser specialist with expertise in treating darker tones, but I urge you to see what the erbium YAG can do for you.

Nonablative Laser Treatments
These nonablative lasers you're reading about (N-Lite, CoolTouch) are marketed as the first and only pain-free way

to improve and erase wrinkles. Much of that is true. There is no pain, no redness, and no downtime after treatment with either of these machines. The laser is designed to pass through the upper layer of skin and head directly for the dermis. The object is to heat the collagen in the dermis (the thick, inner layer of skin) and to stimulate it, causing it to regenerate. Essentially you want to make more collagen. And it works to a degree, but the problem is that sometimes not enough heat is generated to get a tremendously great cosmetic result.

You can expect a positive cosmetic result, but you will need patience. Be prepared to see "nothing at all" at first. Nonablative laser treatments require three months for results to be noticeable, but you will gradually see the wrinkles improve or disappear, a bit or a lot, depending on what you started with. As with other laser treatments, you need to keep up with this, so you will have to repeat the procedure every few months. But there is no down time, no redness, no irritation, and no pain. Nothing but nice skin to follow.

Caveat Emptor!

Anyone who is licensed for medicine and surgery can buy and operate a laser. What this means is that aestheticians who work in hair salons and spas can buy and operate a laser *if*—and this is a Herculean "if"—they are under the supervision of a doctor. The big problem is, what does "supervision" mean? The way the New York State law is written, a nurse or nurse-practitioner or an aesthetician has to be under the supervision of a physician to perform these procedures, but no one has defined what supervision means. In New York it does not mean "on the premises." It means *available by phone.*

That means, if an aesthetician on Thirty-second Street wants to buy a laser and use it, she can call a doctor who may work on Ninety-eighth Street and contract for his "supervision." Then she can split with him some of her income from the procedures. It is very sad, but that's what's going on right now. Florida and New Jersey state laws have disallowed it, however, and hopefully New York will soon follow.

Here's another situation with which I take issue: not only are there few standards as to who can use a laser and who cannot, but perhaps more important, there are few standards as to who can use it on *what*. I'm a dermatologist, but if you ask me to take out your gallbladder using a laser, I'm legally licensed to do it. It's ethically ridiculous. Or, say I'm a gynecologist. I can go out and buy a laser for wrinkles. *Tomorrow*. The technician will come in and train me for an hour, and I'm off and running. That's it. I can put an ad in the *New York Times* saying, "Laser Surgery"; I can even buy a picture of "before and after results" from the company that sells me the laser. Then I can show the before and after pictures and say in my ad, "Look at these two hands I did. Come see me."

So you must be on your guard. If you're considering any laser procedure, ask these questions first:

- *Do you own the laser?* Lasers can be rented. If the laser is rented rather than owned, the chances are, the physician doesn't really use it a lot. Look for someone who owns the laser.

- *Do you have laser training?* If the physician says yes, find out by whom. You want someone who is skilled, not someone who learned at a weekend course. Or worse, someone who was trained by the sales rep. Most of these companies will sell you the laser *and* the training package. And the training package is: the sales representative comes in, you line up a couple of patients for an hour or two, he does a couple with you, you do a couple by yourself, and he says, "Thanks, Doc. I'll buy you dinner." And he's out of there. He's gone. He's on to his next sale. Believe me, using a laser is not that simple. It takes real experience. Make sure anyone you consider letting laser your skin has been doing it for at least six months. There's a learning curve with all these technologies.

- *How many years have you been doing this?* The answer should be "one," at the very least.

- *What is your laser training?* The answer should be "a training course *plus* a preceptorship."

I know. No one asks the questions. Everyone is *afraid* to ask. And even if you do ask, how do you know the answers are legitimate? They may well be, probably are, in fact. But for my money, the best recommendation comes from someone who's already had the procedure done by the doctor you are considering. Before we leave the topic of lasers, let me add here: for 10 percent of patients, lasering doesn't work. In that case we go back to the old chemical peels, TCA (trichloroacetic acid), and glycolic acid, and for those patients, those procedures work. I don't know why, but they work really well.

BOTOX: NOT-SO-SCARY STUFF

Botox, which is short for botulism toxin A, works by affecting nerve endings so that they cannot communicate with certain small muscles, thereby rendering these muscles temporarily inactive. It does not, however, impair sensory perception in the area. Though derived from botulism toxin—a deadly poison—Botox, a purified toxin derived from bacteria, is injected in doses small enough to be harmless. It is, in fact, very, very safe and nowhere near as scary as it sounds.

Used since 1980 for the treatment of strabismus (lazy eye) and blepharospasm (uncontrolled eye blinking), Botox was discovered in the late 1980s to be equally effective on the facial muscles, especially in the forehead and around the eyes, that cause expression lines. Since a 1995 study in the *Journal of the American Academy of Dermatology* demonstrated the substance's power to smooth out frown lines in the forehead, it has become the darling of facial injections, and dermatologists have been struggling to keep up with demand. By way of example, in a given week I can administer up to fifty Botox injections, far outpacing any other single procedure I perform.

The idea behind Botox is simple. If you can relax the muscles whose incessant activity of expression causes furrows to appear, the wrinkles will relax in turn. You may wonder how hindering a normal muscular activity will help your appearance, but keep in mind that the movement you are restraining is hurting your appearance to begin with. When we frown, for instance, we gather the skin between our eyebrows into a fold, producing vertical furrows above the bridge of the nose. In those of us who frown more chronically, these furrows can become permanently etched into the skin, turning an otherwise youthful face into a picture of frustration and anger. It is exactly this predicament that Botox, without surgery or scars, can easily avert.

As with collagen and fat transplants, the effect is temporary, but the procedure can be safely repeated and takes only a few minutes. Botox is quickly injected near the nerves triggering the targeted facial muscle. The area may or may not be immediately massaged to enhance the toxin's reach, and within three to four days—in some cases up to a week—the substance takes effect. Gradually, over three to five months, the paralysis begins to fade, and muscle action fully returns, usually by the sixth month after treatment. When it does, so will the consequent frown lines, but the same simple treatment is all that is needed to get them to disappear again.

Risks

Stories about frozen faces and other disasters of Botox abound, but the truth is that complications associated with this procedure are exceedingly rare. Still, it is advisable to *find a doctor with at least two years' experience with Botox.* The side effects are related to the local injection of the solution, primarily a small chance of a bruise at the injection site, and *never* permanent. In rare cases a loss of sensation occurs in areas of the face not being treated, but again, it doesn't last. Approximately 1 percent of patients will develop a slight lowering, or ptosis, of one eyelid, also temporary and often not even noticeable by the patient. And there is a very slight, but extremely manageable, risk of uneven paralysis, with one area possibly recovering before another.

However minimal the risks, though, it is crucial that Botox, for aesthetic reasons, be injected with moderation and foresight. I feel very strongly that 100 percent smoothness is almost always unwarranted and ill advised, as it will leave the face unsexy and masklike. In most cases I prefer to freeze 80 percent of the muscle instead, which disables it just enough to soften an expression line without compromising your range of expression. Remember, above all else, you want to look natural.

Botox injections cost from $500 to $750 per pair of muscles treated—that is, the left side and corresponding right side.

Related Procedures

Botox will hide most expression lines and keep new ones from forming, but a fat transplant, silicone or collagen injection may also be necessary to even out lines deeply etched into the skin.

Frequently Asked Questions about Botox

Are there any side effects or risks?

Botox, which has been used since 1980 to calm uncontrolled eye blinking and treat "lazy eye," has a very good safety record. And since it is administered with a very small needle, the easy procedure is almost painless and the risk of bruising not severe. It is crucial that Botox be injected in moderation by an experienced dermatologist, as too much "freeze," as we call it, can impart a hardened, plastic look. It is also vital that you not lie down at all for four to six hours after receiving a Botox injection, as the substance can drift to neighboring muscles.

Is there anyone who shouldn't receive Botox injections?
Although there have been no reports of birth defects with the use of Botox by pregnant women or nursing mothers, only limited data are available so far, so I would consider it off-limits to these groups until more data are obtained.

Where is Botox most effective, and where shouldn't it be used?
Botox does its best work on frown lines, specifically the vertical furrows between the eyebrows; paralysis of this area imparts a pleasant, alert look. It is also optimally effective on crow's-feet (the lines jutting out from the outside corners of the eyes) and on neck folds.

For treating the latter, in a procedure that has come to be known as the Botox neck-lift, the substance is injected into the *platysma* muscles, the pair of wide muscles at the side of the neck that draw down the lower lip and the corners of the mouth. As you can imagine, these muscles see a lot of action over the years (they pop out every time you draw down the corners of your mouth in disgust, for example) and eventually emerge from the neck as two loose cords on either side of the chin—a condition known as "turkey neck." A Botox neck-lift works extremely well to keep them in check once they have lost elasticity, producing in some cases face-lift-caliber results.

Botox also works quite well on the horizontal frown lines of the forehead, but this procedure must be done cautiously, as it can cause the brow and eyebrows to droop.

Is there any procedure to permanently disable the facial muscles that cause frown lines?

There is, and it's relatively inexpensive, but it's surgical. It's called corrugator resection, and it involves cutting the same muscles between the eyebrows (the corrugators) that Botox temporarily disables. It's a simple, useful procedure performed under local anesthesia and sedation by a plastic surgeon.

THE FILLERS

Cosmetic filling agents that flesh out wrinkles, spackle smile lines, fill in scars, and plump up lips are not new, but in the last five years they have seen an astonishing surge in demand. The reason is simple: they work. And work well. But take note: the results are generally not permanent.

The benefits of filler techniques—they are precise, affordable, and provide fast results requiring little to no recuperation—are impressive. So routine and effective are these procedures, in fact, that many cosmetic physicians have been known to give themselves a collagen shot or two at the end of a long day. For those of you who have considered plastic surgery or facial resurfacing, it shouldn't be hard to see how a few pinpricks on your lunch hour or on your way home might come as a breezy alternative to a week spent recuperating from other, more invasive procedures. If you don't mind maintaining the results with an occasional "refill," they're positively worth a shot.

Over the decades many substances have been used to fix the age-related soft facial tissue defects that cause wrinkles. Developing the perfect filler has been an arduous and at times frustrating process for the field, and although there is a consensus among practitioners on how an ideal agent should work, so far its manufacture has eluded us. Some fillers have left unfortunate outcomes in their wake and consequently have since been taken off the market. Others, usually due to ephemeral results, have simply failed to pass muster. Nevertheless, we do have some highly effective substances at our disposal, and I will review them here. You'll see that no single type of filler is applicable to every type of wrinkle, but together they form a powerful arsenal for the nonsurgical spot treatment of furrows and folds. While not designed to repair the photoaging-related roughness or blotching that usually accompanies wrinkles, they work below the epidermis to rout wrinkles that resurfacing techniques may fail to reach. As a result, combining a filler procedure with your average laser or chemical peel can make for a powerful one-two punch.

The Animal Fillers: Collagen

You remember that collagen is the vital connective protein that gives the skin its structure, texture, and elasticity. (It is also present in our bones, ligaments, and joints.) Collagen is abundant in young people, and it is why young skin is plump and full-textured. As we age, the collagen in our body becomes depleted. Because its depletion is the biggest cause of wrinkles and sagging skin, the hunt for an effective collagen replacement has been of consuming interest to dermatologists and plastic surgeons.

Although many cosmetic companies might take exception to this, you should be aware that collagen works best when it is injected into the skin, not applied to it in the form of creams or lotions. The most commonly used form of injectable collagen is bovine collagen, which is processed from the hide of a cow. The most popular forms of bovine collagen are Zyderm and Zyplast, water-based compounds manufactured by the Collagen Corporation. Both are easily and precisely controlled and generally well tolerated. Zyderm is used to plump up superficial and medium-depth wrinkles, particularly around the eyes and lips, while Zyplast is used for deeper furrows, as seen in the nasolabial fold. With both substances there is a measurable (around 3 percent) risk of allergy, but the use of skin testing has kept complications to a minimum. When problems do occur, they rarely persist once treatment has been discontinued.

Collagen injections can be slightly painful, but the procedure is mercifully brief, and a fast-acting local anesthesia, typically lidocaine, can be safely mixed in the syringe to minimize discomfort. Before performing collagen enhancement, your physician should closely evaluate your medical history for any contraindications, such as the presence of lupus or other inflammation disorders. If nothing turns up, you're ready for a skin test, which will be performed one month before your scheduled collagen treatment. A small amount of the actual collagen material will be injected into your forearm, observed for the month (for redness, itching, swelling, pain, or even generalized fever), usually followed by a second skin test done along the hairline. During the testing period, your doctor may also have you pretreat the designated area with tretinoin (Retin-A), which promotes collagen production in your fibroblasts and has been shown to improve the overall "take" of the foreign substance. If, a week after the second allergy test, there is no reaction, the procedure can begin.

The Procedure

With an extremely fine needle, a series of small amounts of collagen are deposited directly into the dermis beneath each wrinkle. Each individual prick stings momentarily, but the skin is immediately numbed to the subsequent injections. A cold compress is usually applied after the procedure to reduce swelling. Both Zyderm and Zyplast treatments take fifteen minutes to an hour, depending on the number of areas treated (each site takes ten to fifteen minutes), with good results appearing instantly and lasting usually between three and six months, and in some cases up to a year. Once the collagen begins to break down, however, it reabsorbs into your body and vanishes, and your wrinkles will return.

At the end of the session, the treated area is a bit swollen and remains swollen for six to twelve hours. Although the redness can be easily concealed with makeup, I'd recommend having the procedure done at noon and taking the rest of the day off work. You should also stay out of the sun for about a week. The pinpricks will produce attendant mosquito-bite-like bumps, which fade within two hours. When the lips are treated, swelling and discomfort may persist longer due to their rich vascularity. The risk of allergy having been attenuated, there remains a possibility of bruising or even pinpoint scarring at the injected site, but incidence of either is quite rare. There is also the off chance of developing a late-onset allergy to collagen, which can produce a serious reaction but, again, is not common.

Collagen costs between $350 and $500 per dose, and a dose (1.0–1.5 cubic centimeters) generally covers a set of three or so areas. To get the best results, two treatment sessions scheduled two weeks apart, sometimes requiring more than one syringe, may be recommended. Depending on how long the effects last, all this can get pretty expensive, and if you find yourself "touching up" more than twice a year, you might want to find a procedure that's more cost-effective— silicone, for example. Silicone lasts ten years, requires approximately four treatments for acceptable results, and costs around $500 a treatment. Be mindful that the durability of collagen injections has a lot to do with your doctor's experience with the procedure. Be sure to ask your doctor whether he or she performs the procedure daily, weekly, or monthly—it could make an enormous difference. And by the way, the answer should be "daily" or at least close to that.

Related Procedures

Collagen injections can be performed along with any chemical or laser resurfacing technique, to plump up wrinkles the peels can't reach.

At Face Value

Frequently Asked Questions about Collagen Injections

Are there any side effects or risks?

Collagen is a purified derivative of bovine collagen and is remarkably safe. After the procedure the area will be swollen for six to twelve hours and occasionally may bruise. In 2 percent to 3 percent of patients, there is a risk of allergy, which can set off varying degrees of irritation or swelling, but an allergy test should be conducted before-hand to measure your tolerance for the substance. There is also a small risk of late-onset allergy, but nothing you should be too worried about.

What areas do Zyderm and Zyplast collagen treat best?

Zyderm, which is designed for superficial and medium-depth wrinkles, softens laugh lines in the nasolabial fold, vertical lip lines, glabella lines (between the eyes), horizontal forehead lines, crow's-feet, and acne scars. Zyplast, a thicker substance meant for deeper wrinkles, targets more profound nasolabial furrows and lines in the corners of the mouth and is used to enlarge lips, augment the chin, and accentuate the cheekbones.

How is human collagen filler derived from cowhide?

Actually most collagen in the animal kingdom is essentially identical. What distinguishes human collagen from most other animal collagen is simply an identifying marker, at the end of each protein band, that is specific to each species. Through a special enzymatic process, that end marker is removed, leaving behind a purified, human-ready collagen.

Who should not have collagen therapy?
If you're pregnant, allergic to beef or bovine products, or suffer from an autoimmune or collagen disorder, collagen is not advisable. Consult your doctor.

The Human Fillers:
Autolagen, Dermalogen, and Restylane

Autolagen, otherwise known as autologous collagen or autocollagen, is a collagen filler derived from the patient's own tissue. Although useful when bovine collagen is not tolerated, it is only minimally more effective than its cow-derived counterpart and a lot more time-consuming and expensive, as it must be harvested from the patient and processed before returning it back to the body. And obtaining the requisite tissue involves surgery. If you're going to add that extra step and cost, you might as well opt for autologous fat transplants, a much longer-lasting procedure I'll describe in a moment. However, if you're already undergoing a face-lift or some other procedure in which skin is being removed, storing some autolagen for a later day might make sense.

One of the more recent human-derived collagen fillers is *Dermalogen*, which is made from purified human cells that come from the tissue of human cadavers donated to the Muscular Skeletal Transplant Foundation, a federally accredited agency. Sounds unsavory, but the substance is carefully screened for viruses and sterilized before being shipped to doctors in syringes. Dermalogen, introduced late in 1998 and still awaiting FDA approval at press time, was originally conceived for the 3 percent of the population who are allergic to bovine collagen, but many doctors believe the substance may actually look better and last longer, too. I have not seen enough evidence to back that claim, and in my experience it caused significantly more swelling than traditional collagen, but naturally I am eager for something like Dermalogen to succeed. For now, though, it is fairly rare, and at $650 a pop—double the cost of bovine collagen—I recommend it only to anyone who is allergic to bovine collagen.

On a more positive note, *Restylane*, or hyaluronic acid gel, is a laboratory-made filler I *do* recommend and avidly use. Hyaluronic acid is a gel-like substance found in the space of tissues, the fluid of joints, and the vitreous humor of the eyes, where it acts as an important lubricating and protective agent. In a stabilized gel form that is injected just under the skin using a tiny needle, it has also proved to be an excellent alternative to collagen, adding volume to lips, wrinkles, and facial folds in those areas where depletion of the body's own hyaluronic acid has left the skin brittle and creased. Since it is derived from a naturally occurring chemical, Restylane can be administered immediately, without pretesting for an allergic reaction. Clinical studies have shown that the implanted hyaluronic acid is naturally integrated into the living tissue surrounding it, permitting the free flow of nutritive elements (oxygen and glucose, for example) and allowing dead cells to pass unhindered on their way up to the skin surface. As a result, Restylane has been shown in many cases to produce a healthier, more consistent, and longer-lived result than collagen. It usually lasts between six and nine months but frequently as long as a year. In Europe, as a matter of fact, where it was introduced in 1996, Restylane has largely stolen the spotlight from collagen, and many dermatologists in the United States are already predicting a similar coup here. At a competitively priced $500 per syringe, it's certainly one of the better deals out there.

Fat Transplants: From Here to There

I mentioned earlier that one of the major causes of wrinkles is the loss of subcutaneous fat. Recalling our house analogy from Chapter 1, the fat on which the dermis rests is a vital substructure that naturally slips away over time, causing everything above it to sink. It all starts in our early thirties, when fat loss at the corners of our mouth produces the indentations known, forgive me for this, as "drool lines." This condition worsens over time, drawing these initial lines downward into a "marionette mouth," soon spreading to the lips, cheeks, and just about everywhere else.

Fat can be good, in other words. And the idea behind this procedure is to take fat from where you don't need it and inject it where you do. Doctors began experimenting with the use of fat for soft tissue augmentation over a century ago, but the technique was largely ignored until 1978, when the emerging liposuction craze yielded an abundance of viable fat crying out to be put to some good use. *Autologous* (*from* your own body *to* your own body) fat is easy to implant, seems to correct deeper defects with greater persistence and fewer complications, and is never rejected by your body. By the mid-1980s many dermatologists had come to favor it over bovine collagen for the treatment of an array of aging symptoms. "It's recycling at its best," says one well-known dermatologist of the procedure. If you ask any patient, she's usually thrilled with the "mini-liposuction."

The Process

The fat transplant process involves three distinct stages, with the whole procedure lasting approximately an hour and a half. First, of course, the fat must be harvested, which is to say extracted, from the buttock, thigh, hip, or abdomen, depending on where the fat can be removed with the least disturbance or deformity (although I have yet to meet anyone who doesn't appreciate the mini-liposuction). The donor site is anesthetized with a local anesthetic (usually lidocaine), a tiny incision is made, and with a narrow, tubelike device called a cannula, the fat is suctioned out. Then it is washed in a saline bath to eliminate any impurities. Finally, the fat is placed in a syringe and, in a manner very similar to collagen injections, slowly injected under the skin into the areas where the fat has disappeared, in this case just below the dermis. Unlike collagen, which is injected into the dermis, the superficial layer, fat is injected *under* the skin, or *subcutaneously*. A local anesthetic or nerve block may be used if necessary. From start to finish, the procedure takes about twenty to thirty minutes and causes very little inflammation or discoloration. The possible risks—lumpiness, infection, and bruising—are slight.

While the goal here is not to stuff the treated area, some overcorrection is generally required to compensate for swelling, but because at least half the transplanted fat will be reabsorbed within a week anyway, this tactic never poses a problem. Many doctors remove a year's worth of fat at a time, to be stored in syringes (labeled with your name and Social Security number). These syringes are stored in a freezer (equipped with an alarm to ensure that your fat won't spoil in the event of a power failure) and administered over a series of sessions. It is not known for certain whether this technique is any more successful than having fresh fat extracted with each visit—or whether the fat cells can even survive freezing—but it's definitely more convenient and works very well indeed.

How long does fat transplantation last? As with collagen injections, this is by and large a temporary solution, requiring repeat (perhaps monthly) visits to achieve satisfactory results. However, unlike injectable collagen, which over time is totally reabsorbed, a certain amount of transplanted fat has the potential of developing a blood supply in its new location, thus becoming permanent. In other words, with repeated injections the results will begin to last longer. To be sure, a significant majority of the transferred cells are simply washed away, but studies show that of the approximately 20 percent that come into direct contact with blood vessels in the area, many if not all will make the cut. What's more, even that transplanted fat which is ultimately metabolized tends to stick around several months longer than collagen—up to eighteen months, in fact. And with repeated injections, the results will begin to last even longer.

The cost of harvesting and storing autologous fat ranges from $1,500 to $2,500, depending on the amount extracted. The cost of monthly injections thereafter is around $250.

Related Procedures
Same as with collagen.

Frequently Asked Questions about Fat Transplants
Are there any side effects or risks?
Because the injected fat is harvested from your own body, the risks and side effects are minimal. Bruising or infection can occur at either the harvesting or the injection stage, and there is also the possibility of "lumpy" results, which makes fat transplants a poor option for treating superficial fine lines.

Does the choice of donor site have any effect on the longevity of the results?
A few studies have shown that fat extracted from the thigh, buttock, and abdomen yields better long-term correction, and most dermatologists will choose one of these areas as a donor site. But again, it all depends on where the fat can be most easily removed.

What areas respond best to fat transplantation?
Fat transplants work more effectively on the deeper wrinkles and folds, especially in the forehead, nasolabial fold, chin, and cheeks. But other areas may respond equally well, depending on the shape of your face and the depth of your wrinkles.

Which is better, collagen or fat injections?
There's no easy answer to that question, as some people have had better results with collagen than with fat transplants and vice versa. Some experimentation with the two

procedures may be required to get the best results. But generally speaking, fat transplants are preferred over Zyplast for deep wrinkles because, as I said, some of the transplanted fat is likely to develop its own blood supply and become permanent, while bovine collagen will entirely disappear over time. For superficial and medium-depth wrinkles, however, Zyderm tends to be more cost-effective than fat transplants, which are much more expensive and not ideally suited to repairing smaller defects.

Permanent Fix: Silicone

All of the filler procedures I've described thus far have one thing in common: no matter how well tolerated or effective, they simply don't last. But does that mean they are a big waste of money? Of course not. For many of my patients, the maintenance required to sustain the effects of collagen or a fat transplant is not a bother. After all, the results are generally positive to some significant degree, last up to a year, and repeating the procedure is about as onerous as refilling their car.

I've already reviewed some dramatically effective resurfacing modalities, any of which might offer a long-term solution to a long-term problem. But then, even a laser or chemical peel, while working miracles for the skin's overall texture and vibrancy, can't permanently plump up some of the deeper contours that set in as we age. Short of a face-lift, currently, I think the best procedure is the injection of silicone.

Silicone is an oil—a viscous one—that is injected along the lines of deep wrinkles, expression lines, and acne scars.

The micro droplets of injected silicone cause your own skin cells (fibrocytes) to produce new collagen that replaces lost tissue. A series of injections is required, usually at one- to six-month intervals, to allow new collagen to develop in response to previous injections. The silicone-induced collagen is your own skin's collagen and persists for decades. Maintenance injections at yearly intervals may be helpful to correct further new changes.

Frequently Asked Question about Silicone
Are there any side effects or risks?
Silicone is completely sterile and inert and thus poses no risk of allergic reaction. However, the procedure is fairly tricky and requires a careful, practiced hand, so be sure your dermatologist has performed these techniques with some frequency. With silicone, an improper technique can produce bumps and unevenness. Possible adverse reactions include pain, inflammation, infection, bleeding around the implant, and scarring. The material may also become dislodged or extruded, and there is always a significant risk of inadequate or excessive augmentation.

GIVE YOUR SKIN A JOLT: MESOTHERAPY AND ELECTROSTIMULATION

Mesotherapy

When, several years ago, a team of Parisian dermatologists invited me overseas to introduce me to a procedure called *mesotherapy*—the injection of vitamin complexes directly into the dermis—I was initially skeptical. I knew that the procedure had been performed in France for some thirty-five years, but I had also seen the lackluster effects of countless French topical vitamin creams that had also hailed from that most cosmetically obsessed of countries, so I was not prepared to be blown away. But blown away I was.

After spending several months in Paris familiarizing myself with the technique (with, I admit, some fantastic dining thrown in for good measure), I returned home and became the first U.S. doctor to offer mesotherapy. If I ever had fifteen minutes of fame, this was it. For weeks the phone was ringing off the hook with calls from fashion magazines and dermatological journal editors; even the *New York Times* was interested. And within months mesotherapy had developed a devoted following, with models, TV anchors, and just about everyone else hooked on its simple, affordable, and astonishingly effective formula.

Doctors and beauty experts have been aware for generations of the protective and free-radical-destroying properties of vitamins A, B, C, and E and minerals like zinc and copper. (We will discuss free radicals and antioxidants in detail in Chapter 12, "The Nutrition/Complexion Connection.") But whether the traditional method of taking these vitamins orally can be of much visible benefit to the skin itself is a subject of considerable dispute. After all, when you swallow vitamins, enzymatic juices break them down in your stomach, and there is simply no way to tell the well-meaning little guys to target your skin, hair, or nails.

Does that mean that taking vitamins the old-fashioned way—even those vitamin complexes formulated specifically with skin and hair renewal in mind—will have no effect on your complexion at all? Of course not, but it does mean that ingesting vitamins, while improving the overall health of tissues by shoring them up against environmental assailants, has an inherently diffuse therapeutic effect, helping the body wherever it happens to be deficient. Likewise, even the vitamin-enriched topical patches and creams that have flooded the market in the past few years simply cannot live up to their promises. Why? Well, to quote well-known beauty author Paula Begoun, "You can't put food on your face and have lunch." In other words, the skin being a fiercely protective barrier, topically applied vitamins simply can't penetrate deeply enough to rejuvenate the skin where it really needs it: the cell-generating basal layer and the collagen-packed dermis. What's more, most dermatologists believe that vitamins, because of their chemical instability, deteriorate when added to cosmetic formulas—and aren't, in any event, added to cosmetics in sufficient concentrations to have any effect.

Therein lies the rub, and therein lies the reason the FDA requires that vitamins be called by their chemical names on cosmetics packaging (*tocopherol acetate* versus vitamin A, ascorbic acid versus vitamin C, and so forth)—to prevent people from thinking that topical vitamins are as "nutritional" as the vitamins found in oral supplements or a healthy diet. Yes, there is some evidence that topical vitamin C may provide protection from UV damage, but there is no evidence whatsoever that topical vitamin C or any other topical antioxidant can do anything else to improve your appearance or provide lasting protection against wrinkles. Sorry, folks.

How, then, to feed your skin what it needs where it needs it? Mesotherapy is the answer. It is the most effective, efficient, and logical way of infusing the skin with vitamins and minerals. Cosmetic mesotherapy evolved from anesthetic mesotherapy, an unorthodox method of relieving pain, increasingly popular in Europe, by injecting an ordinary analgesic directly into the painful area. Using a customized "syringe-gun" and a topical anesthetic, the cosmetic version of this technique delivers a quick "cocktail" of vitamins A, B, C, and E, zinc, and copper directly into the skin—just under the surface for fine lines, deeper for more visible creases—in a series of mini-injections with a tiny, 30-gauge needle. The gun punctures the skin in rapid motion, almost like a sewing machine, and the "vitamin cocktail" comes out in tiny droplets under the skin.

Already dubbed "the new collagen," the thirty-minute procedure, generally repeated two weeks later and then every six months thereafter (at about $300 a session), ensures a level of penetration that topical application and oral dosages cannot, and the positive effects are undeniable. Immediately after the procedure, the skin appears supple, hydrated, glowing, and smoother, and unwanted fine lines are less distinguishable. Deeper wrinkles, too, are significantly improved, though the idea behind this procedure is not to peel away damaged skin layers but to help the dermis build new collagen and elastin. In addition, it works to reduce the appearance of acne scars, bolster fragile blood vessels, and help unsightly broken blood vessels heal. Does it eliminate the need to exfoliate or wear sunscreen? No, but as part of a complete skin regimen including religious sun protection, regular cleansing and exfoliation, and as needed, doctor-assisted resurfacing, it will go the extra distance to help you avoid the knife. I highly recommend it.

Electrostimulation

Electrostimulation is another effective means of recharging your skin, only instead of a "vitamin cocktail," your face gets a mixture of ionic and galvanic currents. Sounds a little wacky? It really isn't. It stems from a revolutionary procedure, also widely and successfully performed in Europe, for training weak muscles by using electricity to induce rapid-fire "reps" of muscular activity. As you know, to execute any motion, the brain, through the intermediary of nerves, sends an electric signal to muscles, which respond by kicking into gear. The devices of facial electrostimulation, which generate electrical waves of adjustable frequency and intensity, operate by the same principle. A set of electrodes is fixed on key muscles in the face and neck, which are then gently brought to contract hundreds of times in only a few minutes—without any movement at all. You may ask yourself what the advantage of this type of no-motion "exercise" would be over the traditional facial "workout" you once saw on TV infomercials, a routine that involved actually squinting and assuming other pained expressions before the mirror. Not an invalid question. But remember our discussion of the harmful effects of facial expression from the Botox section. Then take a look in the mirror and squint, and do it again. See the wrinkles you've etched at the corners of your eyes and in your glabella area? While a good idea in theory, as the repeated tightening of your facial muscles might indeed strengthen them to some degree, it will put your skin through the wringer at the same time, accelerating wrinkles rather than preventing them.

With electrostimulation, by contrast, you can strengthen the muscles that lose tone and stretch over the years, improving the skin's foundation without damaging it in the process. In a recent close study of the procedure, in fact, I took masks of twenty-five women before and after electronic stimulation, and the results gave me a pleasant shock: a computerized reading of facial contours showed a 46 percent improvement in visible wrinkling and texture and an average of about a quarter-inch correction in sagging areas. Numerous tests also show that the procedure measurably improves skin circulation, which decreases with age, and reduces muscle tension, which tends to increase with age. Not bad results for an exercise that doesn't require you to move a muscle.

Before you undergo any electronic muscle-stimulation procedure, your physician should closely review your medical history for contraindications, which include epilepsy, most heart conditions, neuromuscular illness, and pregnancy. For electrostimulation to be efficient, you'll likely need a series of sittings over several weeks, each session lasting twenty to thirty minutes at about $300. Between mesotherapy and electrostimulation, mesotherapy is the more popular at my practice, but many of my patients continue to swear by the "current cure"—and it's not difficult to see why.

Related Procedures

Both electrostimulation and mesotherapy work very well to maintain the effects of a chemical or laser peel—or any other full-face cosmetic procedure, for that matter.

Frequently Asked Questions about Mesotherapy and Electrostimulation

Are there any side effects or risks?
The risks of either of these procedures are negligible.

If I'm getting mesotherapy, do I need less vitamins in my diet?
I think you know the answer to that. There is absolutely no substitute for a diet rich in vitamins and minerals and low in saturated fat, and it is no secret that a healthy diet will promote the health of your skin. The skin is in every sense a reflection of your overall health, and what you eat will affect your health and your complexion alike. Nor can you or your skin expect to get all the necessary vitamins from a supplement. Supplements are a good means of rounding out your diet, but they don't approach the benefits of eating fruits and vegetables—and they can't target your skin or any other part of your body. Conversely, mesotherapy does target your skin, but it doesn't do much for your overall constitution. You'll still need to eat well, wear sunscreen, and if your diet isn't sufficiently nutritious, take a vitamin pill.

I've heard that electrostimulation also works well on cellulite. Is that true?
It is true. I'll tell you more about that in Chapter 7, "Legs, Legs, Legs," but electrostimulation does work well to reduce

the appearance of *cutaneous fat* and *hydrolipodystrophy*, a kind way of saying "cottage cheese thighs." The heat breaks up the bands of cellulite. Even better for cellulite, however, is *cellulite mesotherapy*, a technique I developed with a team of French doctors. But, again, more on that in Chapter 7.

four

Tough Customers

The Eyelids, Ears, Neck, Nose, and Chin

By now you are well versed in what certain cosmetic dermatology procedures can do to treat facial aging and convinced, I hope, that surgery is not your only option. In order to paint a complete picture, however, I want to briefly address the isolated facial regions where cosmetic dermatology may not always work wonders. These include the eyelids, the ears, the nose, the chin, and the neck. That is not to say that the techniques discussed in Chapter 3 are of no use on these areas; on the contrary, their role is crucial and should always be considered before opting for surgery. But the fact is that most minor surgeries are also wonderfully effective and safe and in certain cases more likely to achieve dramatic results. Because my goal is to help you do whatever it takes to reverse the ravages of time, wherever and however they occur, I'm not above admitting that the knife is occasionally unavoidable.

To varying degrees, we will all watch our eyelids sag a bit, our earlobes droop a bit, our neck look like, well, our grandmother's. Fortunately, however, these aging signs respond extraordinarily well to a series of opportunities with cosmetic dermatology, aided perhaps by a bit of surgery. I will list them for you here.

EYELIDS

The aging process deeply undermines the structural integrity of that delicate thing known as the eyelid complex. Over time the incessant muscular activity of blinking, squinting, indeed looking, takes a toll on the area's muscular foundation, which, for all its incredible resilience, is still some of the most fragile tissue found in the body. As the upper lids and eyebrows lose elasticity and droop, puffy bags form beneath the eyes, bringing with them a look of constant fatigue. Other areas—such as dark circles, crepy skin, "eye bags," and crow's-feet—also annoy.

Dark circles are an aesthetic result of dark pigment and dilated blood vessels near the surface of the skin. These can be treated—easily and successfully, I might add—with the sweep of a laser. Crow's-feet are erased with the assistance of Botox, as are drooping eyebrows. Done properly, a few shots of Botox in the eyebrow area will lift the eyebrows for a period of four to six months. It's amazing how much younger you will look with just this small procedure. Crepiness under the eye responds well to the laser, if there is not an excess of skin. If you have hollowed-out eyes, we can inject fat or silicone into the area. (See the "Chin" section below for more on the way silicone works.)

It's really the eye bags that are the problem. They are a telling sign of age and, when seen in young people, can make a major difference in how you look and feel about yourself. These bags, or pouches, are fat pads tucked under the thin skin just beneath the eye. In Europe a new medication, called *phosphatidylcholine*, which is essentially a fat-dissolving material, is being injected into fat pads under the eyes, in the neck, and in the love handles to dissolve the fat. The medication is injected in minute doses into the fat pad and dissolves it in a matter of two weeks. The fat gets broken down, goes into the bloodstream, and is urinated out. The drug is FDA approved for oral use in this country as a means of ridding extra fat from the bloodstream but has not yet been FDA approved here for cosmetic purposes. I suspect it will not be all that long before it is.

In any case, if all else fails and bags are not your "bag," you may want to resort to eyelid surgery, which is also known as *blepharoplasty*. In this operation a plastic surgeon removes both skin and fat from the eye area by means of a simple procedure. Incisions are made in existing skin lines in the upper eyelid. Generally a small crescent of crepy skin is removed and the remaining edges of skin pulled together and closed, resulting in a taut upper eyelid. The scars are generally only visible if the eyelid is closed, and in the hands of a good surgeon, not even then. Under the eye the incision is made within a millimeter or less below the eyelash line of the lower eyelids. The fat is removed, the excess skin excised, and the edges closed as above. When the scars heal, they are essentially invisible. Stitches are removed within several days, and the fatty deposits never come back.

EARS

They made fun of you for them back in grade school, and now, just when you've gotten over it, your ears are the biggest and ugliest they've ever been. As you may have discovered, earlobes tend to droop with age, especially if you've worn earrings the size of wind chimes all your life. And because no one thinks to give the ears the same sun protection as the rest of the face, they take a beating over the years, their peachy softness gradually giving way to sun spots and shriveled, dry skin. In men that latter problem is compounded by unwanted hair—as it thins on top, for some cruel reason, it flourishes in the ear, growing in thick, tweezerproof tufts.

Indeed, old-looking ears can be a dead giveaway if you work hard at keeping the rest of you youthful. Happily, though, these problems are a cinch to fix. For wrinkled earlobes I simply laser the earlobes, which gets rid of the wrinkled skin and stimulates collagen so that they puff up a bit as well. To remove age spots, a prescription bleaching cream like HQRA or an ultralight peel with the gentle erbium YAG laser will likely do the trick. Likewise, for unsightly ear hair I recommend the YAG 1064, a quick-pulse laser that is extremely safe and precise and terminates hair for good.

If, however, you have pendulous lobes, you may want to opt for minor surgery known as earlobe reduction, a thirty-minute procedure performed in a plastic surgeon's office, often in conjunction with other facial procedures. Basically the surgeon trims away a crescent-shaped wedge and sutures together the edges of the lobe. After the incisions heal, the scars should be completely unnoticeable.

NECK

The skin of the neck can have several problems attendant to natural skin aging. Like the face, the neck is more vulnerable than some other areas of the body because of its constant exposure to the elements. Similarly your neck may be more bothersome to you because it is equally exposed in your mirror. The sun is the enemy of the neck as much as it is of the face, but few people tend to use daily sunscreen on the neck—because it stains the clothes. As a result, the skin on the neck can become mottled and discolored and can soon sport dark sun spots and broken blood vessels. More distressing for most people, though, is the looseness of the skin, the sagging, whereby the face seems to *melt* into the neck. Not much more fun are the fine wrinkles and the "turkey neck" some of us inherit, which really say "old." Occasionally people get bands around the neck where muscles begin to tighten in certain areas.

Lasering the neck is the way to erase the discolorations, and although the laser wants to make the skin better and thicker, I should warn you that the results are not as great as they are on the face and that the neck is subject to long-term healing. The bands of muscle contraction that circle the neck can be Botoxed with quite good results, but again, the remedy is temporary.

If sagging skin or a crepy neck or the dreaded "turkey wattle" becomes your daily nemesis, the only remedy for this is a surgical face-lift, which is too detailed for me to sufficiently describe here. Suffice it to say, I believe face-lifts are safe and highly effective today, but only, *only* in the hands of a good plastic surgeon. Check credentials (see Chapter 14) and look for patients who preceded you "under the knife" and you should be able to achieve the look you want.

NOSE

The nose poses two problems: its shape and the appearance of the skin that covers it. Like the earlobes, and indeed like much of our skin as we get older, sometimes the tip of the nose has been known to "go south." Skin problems on and around the nose include broken blood vessels, brown spots and large pores, the latter of which can come from aging or as the result of severe acne. The skin across the nose can be lasered or peeled with little trouble and great success. If, however, the shape of your nose is not pleasing to you, a procedure called rhinoplasty is easily available. Rhinoplasty involves refining and changing the underlying structures of the nose to make it smaller or to give it a more pleasing shape overall. Usually the incisions are made though the nostrils, where the scars will remain out of sight. Sharp instruments are used to redesign the nasal bones as well as to shorten or raise the tip of the nose. At the end of the procedure, the skin redrapes over and adheres to the newly designed structure as if nothing had been done.

CHIN

Sometimes even a laser or chemical peel, while working miracles for the skin's overall texture and vibrancy, can't plump up some of the deeper contours that set in as we age. In those cases facial implants are definitely one way to go.

Although a very simple procedure that does not compare to the complexity of a face-lift, we are still talking surgery. Implants are a simple, relatively affordable, and worthy alternative to the more radically reconstructive procedures employed for deep contour correction. Long used to repair traumatic injuries or congenital tissue deficiencies and more recently to cosmetically enhance the chest, buttock, and calf areas, implants are now commonly used in the soft tissue of the face as well. The goal is to augment or highlight the cheeks, tighten the jawline, or redefine the chin. Either in conjunction with a face-lift or skin peel or as a stand-alone operation, the procedure works well to shore up drooping skin, providing a long-term improvement in facial angularity and border definition.

When you think of implants, the first thing that comes to mind may be the silicone implants long used in breast augmentation. Unlike gel- and liquid-filled implants, however, the material used in facial enhancement is a singular substance, a rubbery semisolid not vulnerable to damage or deflation. As a matter of course, any material used in tissue replacement requires FDA clearance. Developing a facial implant that is perfectly malleable as well as safe and stable over time has been a particular challenge, one that dermatologists and plastic surgeons are still hoping to conquer. In the meantime, though, there are so many effective implant substances bearing the government's seal of approval that choosing among them has become a challenge unto itself. From synthetics like Silastic and Proplast to soft tissue or cartilage harvested from your thigh or ear, deciding on the best implant for you requires discernment on your part and sensitive, creative advice from your doctor. Keep in mind that implants, while removable, will ideally become an integral and undetectable part of your living tissue.

FACIAL LIPOSUCTION

Originally developed to treat the torso and thighs, liposuction—the most popular cosmetic technique in the world—has come a long way since making its way to the United States from Italy in the early 1980s. Indeed, the tools of liposuction are now deployed all over the body to remarkable effect, especially under the chin and as an adjunct to face-lifting. Although I do consider all "lipo" techniques properly surgical, albeit minimally invasive, facial liposuction in particular is so simple and effective that I'd be remiss not to include a discussion of it here.

Recall that the idea behind fat transplants is to fill out those areas where the loss of subcutaneous fat has caused the skin of the face to sag. With facial liposuction and a more refined procedure called *microsuction* (the latter pioneered by renowned New York plastic surgeon Gerald Imber), the goal is the opposite: to vacuum away excess facial fat from sagging areas, inducing the skin to "redrape" itself as it heals. A quick, affordable, and pain-free alternative to the face-lift, facial liposuction, like traditional liposuction, permanently removes fat cells using a specially designed steel tube called a cannula, which is inserted into the targeted region through a tiny incision. Whereas in standard liposuction the tube used can be as wide as five millimeters, in the facial procedure it is typically one-third that size, allowing for delicate, controlled suction. The procedure takes about twenty minutes, is performed under local anesthesia with or without sedation, and almost always produces good results. More often the results are excellent.

"Facial lipo" is best for fatty pockets along the jawline and neck, at the corners of the mouth, and below the chin. What's its secret? Well, the truth is, *the procedure works wonders almost by accident.* It seems that drawing out the selected fat from just below the skin's surface leaves the area slightly wounded, prompting it to heal itself and grow tauter in the process. Over the past few years, doctors who regularly perform this procedure have become highly skilled at controlling this abrasion effect, and recent results, in the chin area especially, have been so good as to eliminate the need for fuller surgery. Beyond your late forties, however, your skin will likely not be elastic enough to bounce back on its own. Similarly, if the amount of fat to be removed is substantial, the skin will also probably have lost considerable resiliency. In such cases a surgical resectioning procedure, usually minor, may be needed to achieve the desired effect.

Serious complications with this kind of surgery are uncommon, and the benefits are visible almost immediately. After the procedure your face will be slightly bruised and inflamed for several days, but you'll still look better than you did before, and you should be back to work the next day. Still, I'd recommend having it done on the Friday before a long weekend, which will give you adequate time to heal before resuming normal activity. Within eight weeks your profile will appear dramatically sleeker. When a significant amount of fat must be removed, or when a "minilift" is needed in addition, you can expect to be laid up for seven to ten days, during which you'll be advised to wear a support dressing for most of the day. In that case a complete recovery takes several months.

Facial liposuction is an exceedingly low-risk procedure, but as with any surgery, there is a risk of infection and scarring. However, infection can be all but precluded with preop prophylactic antibiotics, and scars resulting from the technique will be very small and inconspicuous. All facial liposuction patients will experience bruising, which lasts up to three weeks but rarely longer. A certain amount of transient numbness or reduced sensation in the treated area is also common, and there is a very slight chance of permanent numbness resulting from nerve injury. As with any liposuction procedure, the incisions for facial liposuction are made in naturally hidden areas—usually under the chin or behind the earlobes.

five

Blemish Busters

As some of you know, one of the rewards of surviving adolescence isn't, unfortunately, exemption from zits. As a matter of fact, many people who were blessed with blemish-free skin as teenagers can suffer serious breakouts for the first time well into their twenties, thirties, forties, even fifties. And all the angst of being a pimple-faced teen pales in comparison to the anguish of being a pimple-faced grown-up. No one knows exactly what causes decidedly nonteenage skin to break out, but one thing is certain: "late-blooming" acne, which afflicts all skin colors and types, is every bit as distressing as any other aging symptom. Wrinkles alongside zits make for a duo that can destroy just about anyone's self-esteem.

Fortunately, though, adult-onset acne is highly treatable. It may take a bit of experimenting to find the right cure, as no one antiblemish strategy is universally effective, but there is definitely no shortage of tactics from which to choose. But as with wrinkles, you can't fight pimples without understanding the skin conditions that give rise to them.

Even if the myriad factors that spur their formation are not entirely understood, there *is* a clear understanding of how blemishes physically form. First, let's clear up a myth: acne is not about oily skin. You can have the oiliest skin in the world and not have acne. Rather, it's a physiological process that evolves in the pores. Each pore on your face contains a hair follicle that has an oil gland running alongside of it. The oil is shed out the pore and follows up the hair like a little wick. Inside that pore are the tiniest skin cells, epidermal cells that are being sloughed off regularly. In the best of all worlds, the dead skin cells and the oil flow out and are continually shed. What causes pimples to crop up is when the oil glands pump out more oil than can smoothly exit the skin, causing festering bacteria within the pore or follicle to get trapped. Exacerbated by the buildup of hair and skin cells that are also blocked from properly exfoliating, the pore is soon ready to burst. If the pore opens directly on the skin surface, a blackhead—the least unsightly of blemishes—is the result. If a layer of skin covers the top of the pore, however, you have yourself a whitehead, which evolves into a pimple. If the infected blockage occurs deep within the pore, dreaded acne is on its way; and if it's really deep, you are the not-so-proud owner of a cyst.

Why do some of us get acne and not others? Heredity. Pure heredity. Ninety-nine percent heredity. Of course, you can get acne from bad cosmetics, from excessive sweating, even from iodine. But those instances are rare. Ninety-nine percent of acne is yours because your parents had it first.

Most adult acne is cystic. Cystic acne looks different from teenage acne. Rather than having the appearance of small red pustules, cystic acne shows up as larger cysts, which generally occur under the skin and around the jawline. The mechanism is a little bit different, too. It is caused, most often, by stress. Stress stimulates the pituitary gland, the pituitary gland sends a message down to your adrenals, and your adrenals put out some excess hormones. The hormones cause deep clogging of the ducts. Alas, adults also are subject to "teenage acne." What triggers the hormonal imbalance that triggers the sebaceous glands to ruin your skin? Wild hormonal changes being so characteristic of adolescence, it is no surprise that teenagers have it the worst. But keep in mind that hormone levels are volatile at any age, and anything from stress and sun exposure to menstruation can throw them way out of balance.

The important thing to understand is that blemishes grow from the inside out, not the other way around. In other words, while dirt or pore-clogging cosmetics do contribute to blemishes, they are extremely minor factors when compared with hormone-induced oil overactivity. So scrubbing your face five times a day with an abrasive or detergent soap will do little more than leave your skin more irritated than it already is. Likewise the "greasy food" myth. There isn't a lick of solid evidence that acne is actually caused by oily food or that factors like cigarettes or lack of exercise worsen it. True, heavy foods, smoking, and other health destroyers can lead to stress, which has been linked to oil overproduction, but if you're genetically predisposed to acne, will becoming a vegan triathlete solve your problem? Doubtful. Of course, if you notice that cutting something out of your diet or exercising more often helps your acne, by all means do so. For most people with serious acne, though, the answer will simply be: get help.

Before choosing an acne strategy, the first thing you must know is that most over-the-counter blemish "cure-alls" are bogus. They may control acne, perhaps, but will not cure it. The word *cure* means you take a pill or use a cream and it doesn't come back. Only Accutane does that. I won't name names here, but I will stress the importance of comprehending the exact causes of blemishes before emptying your wallet at the cosmetics counter.

As with wrinkles or sun spots, you cannot expect to rid your body of pimples (otherwise known as zits) without fully evaluating and fully reversing the things you might be doing to worsen them. Keep in mind that because pimples are the combined result of oil gland overactivity and the buildup of both bacteria and dead skin cells in the pore—and nothing else—any effective strategy for getting rid of them must do one of three things. The first is *disinfecting the skin*, keeping the pores clear of the bacterial goo that causes it to become inflamed. The second is *exfoliating*, or prompting dead skin cells to float to the surface and shed at a healthy clip. Because aggressive exfoliation also runs the risk of aggravating acne, however, you must learn the delicate art of encouraging cell turnover without irritating the skin. Finally, your blemish plan of attack must include a strategy for *keeping your oil glands in check*. At the least this will mean avoiding greasy products that keep excess sebum from flowing out of the pores. In tougher cases it will mean taking a prescription drug that actually shrinks or otherwise stifles the sebaceous glands.

RULES FOR DEALING WITH BLEMISHES

The following general rules should help you to put your blemish disorder in perspective and choose a plan of attack that works for you.

Rule 1: Don't Run to a Dermatologist as Soon as You See a Few Pimples

Unless you have a serious condition, your doctor will likely recommend an over-the-counter soap or ointment containing none other than *benzyl peroxide*, to be used with the ubiquitous exfoliant *salicylic acid.* Benzyl peroxide, which is available in much gentler formulations (of 2.5 percent, 5 percent, and 10 percent) than when you were a teenager, is a tremendously effective antibacterial agent that, when combined with (1 percent to 2 percent) salicylic acid, will do the trick for most late-blooming pimple sufferers. You don't need a doctor to tell you what's available at the local drugstore, and you have nothing to lose by starting there first.

If you are one of those insomniacs who watch *acne infomercials* instead of counting sheep, and if you start to wonder what miracles *those* hyped products contain, forget it. All those products are glycolic acid and benzyl peroxide, which you can buy over the counter. Benzyl peroxide can be purchased by prescription or over the counter with absolutely no difference except price. Salicylic acid also can be purchased over the counter. Salicylic acid is a derivative of aspirin that comes in a cream. And guess what? This cream is known as *beta hydroxy.* That's right. Beta hydroxy, the "ultimate" newest of new beauty creams hyped all over the media, is just pure salicylic acid. The very same salicylic acid and benzyl peroxide that you see on infomercials and in prescription drug advertisements can be found in many products readily available on the drugstore shelf. Take a stroll down the drugstore aisles and read a few labels. Propa pH is based around salicylic acid. Clearasil and Stridex are based around benzyl peroxide. Neutrogena is based around salicylic acid and contains a little benzyl peroxide. So why pay the extra money?

Caveat Emptor!

Most of these medications are for teenage acne. They do dry up the skin and exfoliate it, and in so doing, they dry up the pimples and heal them. No secret there. But one of the problems with adult *cystic* acne is that everybody goes to the drugstore and buys teenage medications to treat it. If they don't work, and they probably won't, the next step is to use a topical antibiotic like *erythromycin, tetracycline, clindamycin,* or some generally effective combination of erythromycin and *zinc acetate* or erythromycin and benzyl peroxide. The latest is a clindamycin and benzyl peroxide combination. Topical antibiotics take longer to work but also carry fewer side effects than oral antibiotics, which can cause indigestion and vaginal infections and yellow the teeth, among other complications.

When topical antibiotics fail to do the job, oral antibiotics, like the tetracycline family, are a good option, provided you consider the drawbacks carefully. Keep in mind that *oral antibiotics kill a lot of good bacteria along with the bacteria causing you harm and that after a while your body is likely to adapt to them, making them completely useless.*

For severe acne you may want to consider Accutane. This powerful drug, like tretinoin, is derived from vitamin A. It works, and works extremely well, by shrinking the sebaceous glands, in turn smothering oil production. Once used only for cystic acne, it is now widely prescribed for milder cases of acne when traditional treatments fall short. Because it carries serious side effects, however, its popularity has come with considerable controversy.

I'll tell you the bad news first. Chief among Accutane's side effects is that it can cause serious birth defects in developing fetuses—90 percent of the time, according to one major study. So if you're pregnant or are trying to get pregnant, don't even go near the stuff. If you're not, however, using a condom or a diaphragm isn't going to cut it: you'll need to take a birth-control pill. In other words, there cannot be even the remotest possibility that you will conceive while taking the drug, and after stopping treatment, you should talk to your physician about how long you should wait before discontinuing birth control.

Those of you who aren't pregnant, though, may still face certain significant side effects with Accutane, including dry, itchy, red, peeling skin; irritated eyelids, eyes, and lips; mild nosebleeds; some hair loss; indigestion and nausea; and mood swings. The majority of Accutane users suffer few, if any, of these symptoms, however, and the number of people who actually have to stop treatment due to side effects is negligible.

Now the good news. Accutane is the most effective drug for acne that I have ever seen. Not only does a typical four-month treatment radically shrink oil glands, putting the squeeze on the sebum that generates breakouts, but also in many cases it shrinks them permanently—reducing full-blown acne to nothing more than the occasional pimple for the rest of your life. In those cases in which acne recurs following Accutane therapy, the condition tends to be far less serious the second time around and often responds well to less powerful medications.

As for the possible side effects, there are simple things you can do while taking the drug to ease discomfort. A light moisturizer for sensitive skin will soothe dryness and irritation. For dry eyes try artificial tears. Check with your doctor, but temporarily discontinue tretinoin or AHA therapy. If you experience mood swings, chalk them up to the drug.

Rule 2: Don't Single Out Zits

Once a blemish has reared its head, there is little you can do to zap it away, although commercials featuring teenagers who have never had a pimple in their lives tend to imply otherwise. This means that merely smothering your three zits in benzyl peroxide will only irritate an already irritated area and do nothing for the areas where blemishes might form next. *Always consider your whole face when you are cleansing or applying an antibacterial ointment. The key is prevention, not annihilation.*

Rule 3: Don't Scrub, Scrape, Squeeze, or Pick

Most people know that popping zits, hugely gratifying though it may be, causes your face to become pitted and scarred. Not to mention the fact that it spreads bacteria-

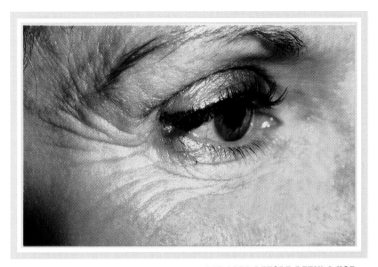

EYE AREA BEFORE RETIN A USE

This woman's deep smile lines came from many happy days (and too much sun). She felt they belied her age, however.

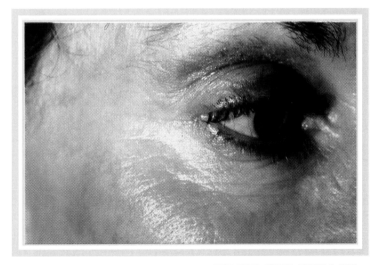

EYE AREA AFTER RETIN A USE

Here they have been dramatically reduced, thanks to diligent use of Retin A.

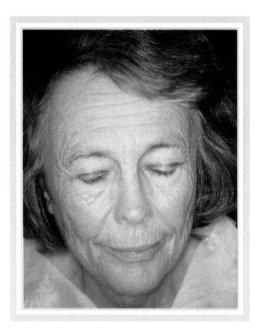

BEFORE CHEMICAL PEEL

Too much time on the tennis court for this patient.

AFTER CHEMICAL PEEL

The results of a deep chemical peel have taken at least fifteen years off her face. She was and still is thrilled with the outcome.

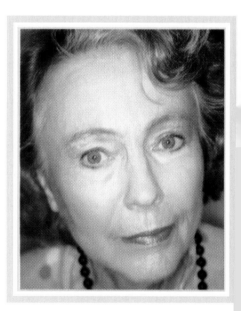

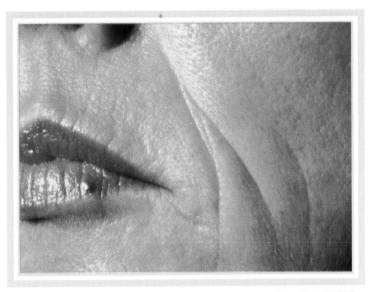

LIPS BEFORE COLLAGEN TREATMENT

One more reason not to smoke. The deep lines are also a result of natural fat loss that comes over time.

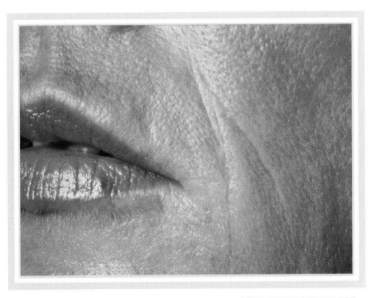

LIPS AFTER TREATMENT

Her lips and the surrounding area are now plumped out like they were ten years ago. (All the smoker's pucker lines are evened out.)

HAND WITH PROMINENT VEINS

This woman has thin skin, which
led to these prominent veins.

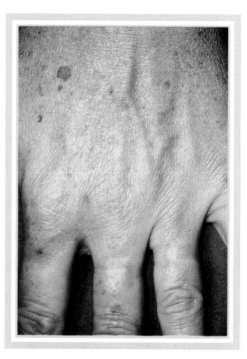

HAND AFTER VEIN TREATMENT

With the veins almost totally diminished, her hands now match
her youthful face.

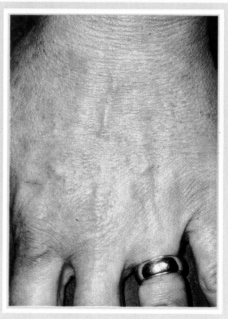

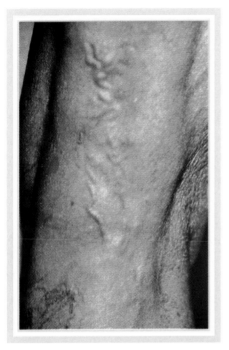

LEG WITH VARICOSE VEINS

This patient has heredity to thank for these varicose veins, but I suspect she also may have spent too many days on the beach in the Bahamas.

LEG WITH VEINS TREATED

"Look, Ma, no veins." (It looks very smooth.)

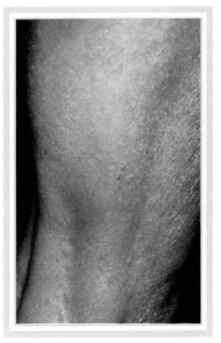

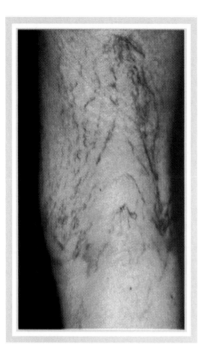

LEG WITH SPIDER VEINS

These are also hereditary and can come at any age, adding years to your legs.

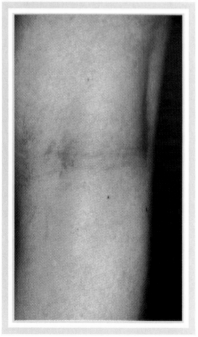

LEG AFTER SPIDER VEIN TREATMENT

These legs look smoother and naturally younger.

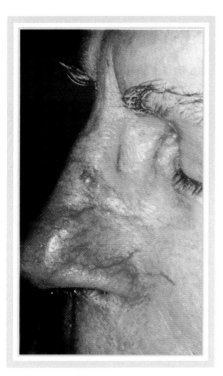

MAN'S FACE WITH ROSACEA

The nose is very red and looks like it has red broken veins. This man has rosacea and hated that his nose always appeared so red.

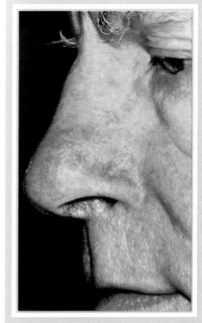

MAN'S FACE AFTER ROSACEA TREATMENT

He was delighted that we could get rid of so much of the redness.

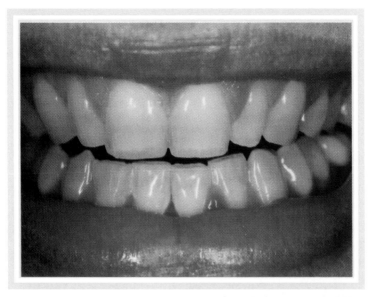

TEETH BEFORE PORCELAIN LAMINATES

Who among us couldn't use brighter, straighter teeth?

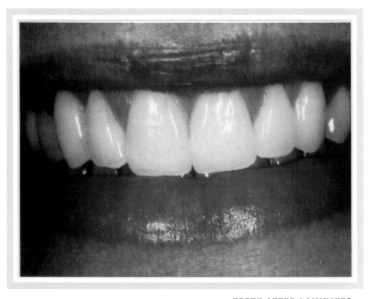

TEETH AFTER LAMINATES

The laminates have made her teeth look brighter, straighter, and more uniform in size.

ridden sebum to surrounding areas and to your fingers, leading to more breakouts in a hurry. A lesser-known upshot of squeezing blemishes, furthermore, is that it wreaks havoc below the surface, especially on collagen. Every time you pinch, you stretch out your skin's elastic foundation, accelerating wrinkles. It's a bad idea all around.

Rule 4: If You Have Acne, Don't Moisturize with Heavy Creams

For acne sufferers moisturizers are bad news indeed. Why? In a word, they clog pores, regardless of whether they're "oil-free." After all, a moisturizer is by definition designed to replicate the effects of sebum, which, in normal supply, keeps the skin and hair healthy. So if excess sebum is your problem, slathering on a sebum substitute is obviously not a good idea. And while "oil-free" moisturizers, which contain substances like triglycerides or plant waxes and claim to be noncomedogenic (meaning they won't block pores), are considerably less "greasy," they still contain pore-stuffing, acne-inducing ingredients. As a matter of fact, most "oil-free" moisturizers are even more likely to clog pores than their petrolatum-based counterparts. The same goes for waxy "oil-free" makeup. In cases in which acne crops up alongside exceedingly dry skin, resist the temptation to use moisturizer on isolated parched patches. Instead, try to figure out what other ingredients in your antiacne arsenal might be causing the imbalance.

Rule 5: Clean the Skin Carefully

On broken-out skin, it is critically important to use a nonabrasive, water-soluble cleanser. It is also vital to use tepid rather than hot water (which is believed to "steam" the face and open up clogged pores but in actuality burns the face, causing irritation and further oiliness). Cetaphil Skin Cleanser is one excellent product, but there are a number of good facial washes out there. Neutrogena is good, and so are Propa pH and Clinique. Almost every beauty product line makes one. Feel free to experiment to find one that pleases your skin. Two golden rules, however: One, *don't use anything that comes in bar form.* To stay solid, bar soap must contain a host of waxy thickening agents that, like tallow, clog pores. And two, *if you feel inclined to try a mild abrasive designed for acne sufferers, go at it gently;* the rougher you are, the more aggravated your oil glands may become. The same goes for taking off makeup—don't wipe or scrub it off, which will abrade and stretch out your skin and jam your pores. This is true especially for lipstick: while lips are pore-less and immune to breakouts, the skin surrounding your mouth is as prone to breakouts as any other part of your face, so be sure to apply and remove your glosses carefully.

Many people have been wondering about Bioré Pore Perfect Deep Cleansing Strips, which are sold at drugstores everywhere. These superadhesive strips of cloth, which are placed over the bridge of the nose and, some minutes later, yanked off, claim to pull blackheads out from the root (along with some superficial skin), but do they work? Since they're not expensive (about a dollar apiece), and a lot of my patients do swear by them, I say, "If you want to, why not?" But I warn you: *it's a bit of a striptease, so don't get hooked.* After you rip off a Bioré strip, you will be pleased to see how much gunk it has actually taken with it. But the truth is that, in this fashion, there is no way to pull out anything but the tip of the blackhead, leaving the rest of the ugly thing intact. With regular use, some tell me that they've gotten their pores noticeably clearer, but many dermatologists are concerned about the safety of daily stripping. There is a reason, after all, the manufacturer itself warns against using the product on dry or sunburned skin. I would also recommend not using these strips if you are using tretinoin or AHAs.

Rule 6: Exfoliate

We've already discussed the importance of daily exfoliation in your fight against wrinkles. The added burden of late-blooming acne gives you all the more reason to get started. For either condition the exfoliating agents are much the same, so little adjustment to your antiaging regimen is required. I'd recommend trying a six-month course of 7 percent to 8 percent nonemollient-based alpha hydroxy acid every morning and Retin-A (in this case cream-based) every night. Used together, AHAs and tretinoin are capable of remarkable feats. Some, however, have had better results from using azelaic acid or Differin instead of Retin-A. Azelaic acid, a saturated dicarboxylic acid derived from wheat and barley, is a powerful exfoliant that disinfects at the same time. Commonly known as adapalene, Differin is a very good

topical retinoid made by Galderma, the company that makes
Cetaphil. It is said to be far less irritating than tretinoin, and
one recent study in the *Journal of the American Academy of
Dermatology* claimed it was more effective on acne, too. Still,
I would try Retin-A first, see how well you tolerate it, and
go with Differin (which, like Retin-A, requires a prescription) only if tretinoin leaves your face extremely irritated.

Rule 7: Try a Laser Acne Peel

For some cases of tough acne, I used to recommend a
series of medically performed alpha hydroxy acid peels,
which use concentrations of up to 70 percent to dissolve the
stratum corneum, followed by a milder AHA preparation to
be applied at home, sometimes in tandem with tretinoin.
That worked well, but not as well as my latest all-purpose
tool: the erbium YAG laser. A ten-minute procedure safe
enough to be repeated every six weeks, the erbium YAG
laser facial exfoliates the skin much more gently and precisely than a fruit-acid peel (or previous lasers, for that matter), taking out blackheads and whiteheads along the way.
See the "Laser Resurfacing" section in Chapter 3 for details
on this remarkable laser.

Rule 8: Keep Wearing Sunscreen

Wearing sunscreen is a bit tricky, I admit, as even oil-free
sunscreens are capable of clogging pores, but you still need
to find a way. Try experimenting with sunscreens that are
made for oily skin (in a nonmoisturizing base, that is). If you

find one that doesn't make your acne worse, stick with it. But remember, it must offer both UVA and UVB protection to be worthwhile.

ROSACEA

Rosacea is a chronic condition that shows up as a general redness on the face, mostly across the cheeks but also occasionally on the forehead and chin. The skin across the area may become dry and eventually give rise to pimples. These pimples look like teenage acne, but they don't have the blackheads or whiteheads that are attendant upon teenage acne. In fact, because of the similarity, rosacea has been called "adult acne." Rosacea is caused by flushing, which occurs when, for some reason, a large amount of blood flows through the normally tiny, unnoticeable blood vessels close to the skin's surface. When this happens, the vessels dilate to handle the flow, the valves break, and the vessels become permanently dilated. Once blood flow to the skin is increased, that increases oil production by the oil glands, resulting in a kind of acne as well as redness, itchiness, and scaliness. As the vessels get larger, and because they are directly beneath the skin, the redness becomes more apparent. At first the enlarged blood vessels look like thin red lines on the face, called telangiectasias. In truth, no one really knows what causes this condition.

There are several ways of treating rosacea. You can use topical creams or oral antibiotics, or you can use a laser. Topically you use either steroids or metroconizole creams. Antibiotics include tetracycline or a derivative. But these creams and antibiotics only treat the symptoms; they don't treat the dilated blood vessels.

At this particular time, the only way I know to treat the underlying physiological problem is with a 532 Medlite laser, which is used to destroy the dilated blood vessels. Behind the poorly working blood vessels is a new bed of capillaries with blood vessels that are still microscopic and still working perfectly. If those vessels are going to dilate and become rosacea, and they probably will, it will take years before that happens. So the rosacea improves. The laser has treated the underlying problem, so you need less creams, less tetracycline, plus you flush less and you look better. That's the trick to treating rosacea. You are *fixing* the broken plumbing rather than merely putting patches on it.

six

Gloves Off!

Recently I was working out on a treadmill in Miami, and who should be on the machine next to mine but Dyan Cannon—that gorgeous star of movie fame (and one-time wife of Cary Grant)—who looked, I must say, remarkable. She had a young face, young attitude, great energy. In fact, every *pore* on this woman spelled *young*—until, that is, she grabbed a towel in her hand and put it to her brow. And that, as they say, was the killer. The difference between her face and her hands was twenty years! Bottom line? You can look absolutely spectacular, but if you want to fool the world about your age, you've got to consider your hands. Fortunately many techniques are available today to keep hands looking young—all of which are safe *and* effective. And no one, believe me, will ever say, "Oh, look! She's had her hands done."

HOW HANDS AGE

Like the skin everywhere else on our body, the skin on our hands is composed of a layer of fat, on top of which lies a layer of dermis, and on top of that the outer layer of epidermis. Interspersed within these layers is a system of blood vessels. As we age, the same thing happens to our hands as to our faces: the fat dissipates, the dermis shrinks, and the outer layer of skin, the epidermis, becomes discolored by brown spots, thinner, and less organized. But what you see on your hands that (thankfully) you won't see on your face is a natural protrusion of veins you never knew existed. If you're wondering where, all of a sudden, they came from, you should know that these veins have been there all along. It's just that with time they may have become larger, the skin overlaying them thinner, the fat dissipated, and, well, there they are.

The skin on the hands differs from that on the face. Hand skin is more like the skin on your forehead. That's because, like the forehead, the hands are bony. So the hand skin sits mostly on a bony prominence. There is no big layer of fat or muscles there to start with, either. Rather, the muscles are quite fine, like those you find in the forehead.

Before we get to the procedures, you should know that *the skin on the hands does not heal as quickly as the skin on the face.* As a result, everything we do on the hands takes up to two to four times as long to heal. The face heals unbelievably quickly—it's so forgiving—but the hands, unfortunately, are not. There's an old saying in medicine: The farther you get away from the heart, the slower the healing. There's no scientific data behind this, except anecdotally, but if you watch, you'll see: the hands heal slower, and the feet heal the slowest.

So what's the secret to keeping your hands looking as young as possible? Several things. None of them a secret. Prominent veins can be remedied with a procedure called vein *sclerotherapy*. For skin that appears loose due to diminishing fat, we inject fillers, and for brown spots and discolorations, the answer is *laser peels, chemical peels, bleach,* and *sunscreen*. None of these therapies is perfect, mind you, but many are quite acceptable. I'm going to address them all here because they are still used in different areas across the country. I don't use them all, though, and I will tell you my honest opinion of their efficacy. Of course, the optimal care for hands is identical to that for the face and can be summed up with an old adage: "The best offense is a good defense." In other words, if you want to do your hands, and yourself, a favor, remember the three little words: sunscreen, protection, and hydration.

REDUCING PROMINENT VEINS

Now for the procedures. Let's start with the problem of protruding veins. As I said earlier, the thinner the skin and the less fat on the back of the hand, the more likely the veins will protrude, producing a telltale, age-revealing ropy effect. The approaches that work best to reduce the prominence of—or to destroy—these veins are the injection of sclerosing agents, the laser, the addition of fat, or all three.

Sclerosing

To sclerose (shut down) a vein is a fairly simple procedure that involves injecting a saline (saltwater) solution or some other agent that encourages inflammation directly into the vein. The irritation causes the vein to collapse, and the collapsed vein generally seals itself off. Ultimately the body absorbs the nonviable tissue, and you'll never know there was once a vein there. This procedure is used for the veins of the lower extremities as well and for the same purpose. People worry about "giving up" a vein, believing that every vein in the body is necessary. This is far from true, though. The important veins, the ones that function as a pathway for blood as it returns to the heart, lie deeper within the musculature. The veins we're talking about sclerosing, those closest to the skin, are called *superficial veins* because they are really not that important.

The heart pumps oxygenated blood into the arteries, which carry it around the body. The arteries radiate out into the body, just like the branches of a tree, getting smaller as they move farther away from the heart. Eventually, as they reach up to the skin, they get increasingly narrow and ultimately become capillaries—small bundles of blood vessels. In the capillary complex, there is a transfer of heat, nutrients, and oxygen to and from the skin. It is here, too, that the veins pick up the depleted blood and return it to the heart. Blood depleted of oxygen is bluish in color, which is why the veins in the hands and legs appear blue. Every vein throughout the body contains valves, which keep the blood flowing in the right direction (back toward the heart). But when a valve weakens, which it can just from the natural process of aging, the blood backs up into the vein. The pressure from the increased blood supply against the walls of the vein causes it to dilate; hence, the appearance of veins on older hands.

HEALING

After sclerotherapy the veins and their surrounding area can turn black-and-blue almost overnight and can remain this way for several weeks to months. Yes, months. Many women are willing to put up with discoloration for a week, but a month? Not likely. If you sclerose your hand veins, be prepared to look as if you had just gone a round with "Rocky." Though you might not pack his punch, you *will* be able to use your hands right away. And there are, of course, different types of camouflage makeup you can use while healing, many of which work quite well. But most women reject the idea of using them. At least they have never caught on with *my* patients.

Fillers

Another option for hiding the veins is to plump up the layers beneath the skin so the veins will appear less prominent. Additionally the skin will look less wrinkled. *Fat, collagen*, and *silicone* have all been used on the backs of the hands for this purpose. In fact, any filler that can be used on the face can be used on the hands. As with the face, we inject these substances under the skin. I don't consider it the best option for the hands, however, because hands are always in motion. They're constantly stretching and bending and lifting and rubbing against things, and the endless movement tends to break down the fillers a lot more quickly than the fillers in the face break down. So I can inject all I want; it's not going to last that long. Also, as far as I'm concerned, it's hard to get fat, or any of the other fillers (silicone and collagen included) to lie smoothly on the backs of the hands. In my practice I have not had much success with fillers, and I rarely use them unless a patient insists.

If you choose to use fat as a filler, it will generally come from your hip area and will be removed by a process known as mini-liposuction. The drawn-off fat is processed in the syringe and immediately injected under the skin in several places. The procedure produces swelling for a week or so. Sometimes the needle will hit a vein and that may cause bruised-looking hands for two weeks. Again, it's a very easy procedure to do, but it's not easy to get the look uniform. I have also found that these types of fillers don't last that long. I am much more in favor of *mesotherapy.*

Mesotherapy

Mesotherapy is the equivalent of receiving vitamin injections into the hands. The mixture of a scientific combination of vitamins C, A, E, and the minerals zinc and copper is injected in microdroplets into the skin on the back of the hand using a special needle gun. The object is to regenerate collagen and elastin while also plumping up the skin. (It plumps up the skin by stimulating tissue growth.)

As I discussed in Chapter 3, mesotherapy works quite well, and this goes for the hands as well as the face. Because this vitamin and mineral mixture basically helps the skin generate new collagen and new elastin tissue, the results are not only plumper skin but thicker and younger-looking skin as well. And what's more, mesotherapy helps the epidermis reorganize so it looks brighter. I find it much more effective than trying every day to rub on the equivalent in creams. Creams don't always get absorbed as you'd want them to, so the benefit is going to be different. You'll get a 100 percent benefit with mesotherapy versus 20 percent with cream.

ATTENDING TO BROWN SPOTS

Brown spots, another age revealer, are commonly known by that most inappropriate of names: *liver spots*. Some call them sun spots or age spots. I prefer to call them by their medical name, which is *lentigines*. In any case they are caused, quite simply, by a proliferation of melanocytes in the skin. You will recall from Chapter 1 that melanocytes are the cells that manufacture melanin, the dark pigment in the skin. Most of us have some type of pigmented lesions, including freckles and lentigines, which generally arise as a result of excessive sun exposure, aging, pregnancy, and in response to some medications such as birth-control pills. They're hard as anything to get rid of, I might add. But we *can* get rid of them with nonsurgical procedures, including chemical peels, bleaching creams, and lasering.

Chemical Peeling with Trichloroacetic Acid

We know from Chapter 1 that the skin's pigment cells, the melanocytes, sit directly between the epidermis and the dermis. If you peel off the epidermal cells with a chemical, like trichloroacetic acid, and do it using the proper concentration, in one or two treatments, usually one, you can generally wipe away all the brown spots. The problem is, not only do the brown spots go, but you denature everything—the brown spots, the melanocytes, the epidermis. *Everything*. And so everything has to regenerate. And with this procedure, there's some potential for scarring, because it's not specific only to the brown spots. It also affects the normal skin. And here's the rub: it doesn't always work. Understand, too, that in any case, no matter what you use, you have to use bleach for maintenance—that is, to keep the melanocytes turned off so more brown spots won't arise. Plus, you have to use sunscreen, of course.

Chemical Peeling with Retin-A

Chemical peeling with a Retin-A derivative works on two levels. First, it exfoliates—that is, peels off—the outer layer of skin on the back of the hand, which stimulates the growing cells and results in a new, younger-looking layer of skin. On a second level, the vitamin A derivative appears to work somehow on the skin to entice it to grow new blood vessels, collagen, and elastic tissue.

The process of exfoliation is similar to what happens when men shave. Because I shave every day, I am mechanically stripping my outer layer of skin every day. And every day I send a message to my growing layer of skin to regenerate. That's why in two people of equal age, a man and a woman, the man's skin looks younger than the woman's does. It's daily exfoliation. Which is what Retin-A does. It exfoliates the skin on a daily basis, microscopically, and as it does so, it sends a special signal to the growing layer of skin, stimulating it to perk up and increase the metabolism. The result is younger, thicker, better-textured skin.

The downside of Retin-A is that it's irritating, and most people don't use it daily as prescribed. They get a little irritation, and they stop and wait till the irritation goes away. So maybe they'll use it once a week. How good is once a week? No one knows. In all the studies it's used regularly—the researchers get the patients in the study through the terrible drying-out period, which lasts from eight to twelve weeks.

If you are religious with Retin-A and get rid of your sun spots and are diligent with sunscreen, will you never have spots again? I don't know. Unfortunately *there is no perfect sunscreen*. Still, if you're diligent, and especially if you use zinc oxide, which is the only *total* sun block, it would take a long time for them to come back.

Laser Treatments

For brown spots I much prefer to use a laser because it's so much more specific than any of the other methods. It hits the target and *only* the target. Lasers can scar, too, but that occurs less than 1 percent of the time. You may get a white scar, or it may be a raised, hypertrophic scar, but if you jump in right away, it's fixable. As for healing time, compared to a laser, the chemical peel takes twice as long.

Lasers work extremely well for getting rid of brown spots on both the face and the hands. Today's lasers are tuned to be picked up only by specific colors, so they're not destructive to any of the unaffected surrounding tissue. For example, if a laser is tuned for brown (as in brown spots), the brown pigment is the *only* area on the skin's canvas that picks up the laser's energy. If that same laser tuned for brown were pointed at the hand of a baby whose skin is light pink, nothing would happen.

Sixteen years ago I got my first laser, and it picked up everything in sight. But today lasers have become very target-specific and highly selective. As the wavelengths become more and more precise, they can be programmed to hit just what you aim for—not just brown, for example, but reddish brown, and not just reddish brown but a certain *shade* of reddish brown. Only that shade picks up the wavelength. That's why lasers are so good—they don't damage surrounding tissue.

We use a 532 Medlite laser for sun spots on the body because it's geared to be picked up by colors. It's basically foolproof. As for how it feels, at worst it feels hot. Some people liken it to a rubber band's being snapped against their wrist. The darker the brown, the more energy picked up; the more energy, the more heat; the more heat required, the more it stings. But I always use a numbing cream first and rarely get a complaint. What you're left with after a treatment to the back of the hands is a series of purple dots, which fade, along with the spots, in a week or two.

Some people are so taken with this procedure, they don't know where to stop. Where *do* you stop? You can do the hands, the forearms, the arms, the shoulders, and the back. These places always have some hyperpigmented lesions. So do many women's chests just under the neck. Some men and women do the whole area at a single sitting.

You have to target each lesion specifically. For me to do an individual lesion takes two seconds with a laser that pulses ten times a second. I can cover an arm with perhaps a hundred lesions in fifteen minutes. The most important part of the laser is not only what kind of laser you use but how you set it. Lasers are tunable in all different strengths. Another important aspect of the treatment is who does it. Remember what I said in Chapter 3: experience is a big thing here, and it matters a lot.

Bleaching Creams

I have discussed bleaching creams in depth in Chapter 3. The creams work identically on the face and hands. But I'd like to reiterate that bleaches can be a bit tricky and require a good amount of patience. Bleach takes a long time to fade brown spots—forever, in some cases. Even with the addition of Renova, the best bleaches in the world will not work 100 percent.

OK, I'll amend that. If you use the right amount of bleach—a 4 percent hydroquinone—the right amount of retinoic acid (.05 percent), and you really do it every day, in a year's time you'll probably erase the spots. Probably. But again, it's very hard to stick to a schedule like that. Which is why we combine bleaches with lasers.

In any case, to maintain it all, you're going to have to bleach your hands the rest of your life, because you want to keep the pigment-producing cells, the melanocytes, turned off. So keep using the bleach once or twice a week, or use a hand cream with bleach. And, of course, sunscreen.

Sunscreens

Sunscreens are important, and we'll discuss them in depth in Chapter 10, but as regards the hands, you should know the importance of applying and *reapplying* sunscreen. Think about it. You're always doing something with your hands. And so the sunscreen is getting wiped off all the time. If it's not there, it can't work. Simple as that. If you don't think the sun does terrible damage, just look at the hands of a golfer. One hand looks great—the gloved hand—and the other looks terrible. Sun damage, pure and simple. Golfers are notorious for not wearing sunscreen because it affects the grips on the golf clubs. They say it ruins them. Boaters won't wear sunscreen because they say it stains the teak in the wood on boats. To each his own. I can only say once again, we're fortunate to have so many tools at our disposal to keep our hands looking great, but you have to remember to use them. In other words, to repeat what I said at the beginning of this chapter: *If you want everyone to forget your age, don't forget your hands.*

seven

Legs, Legs, Legs

This chapter corresponds to the previous one, with a few new procedures thrown in for good measure. Whereas the chapter on the hands concerned veins and sun spots, here we will turn our attention again to veins, but now we're looking at both spider and varicose veins. We will also explore the options for getting rid of that puckered, dimply skin on the thighs, hips, and buttocks—that scourge of women around the world: *cellulite!*

UNSIGHTLY VEINS

Road maps! Could there be a *less* flattering description—or a more accurate one? You know what I'm referring to. Those red and purple highways that course in clusters across the once-unblemished landscape of your legs, reminding you that you're not twenty-one anymore. For some reason these thin little veins appear only on the surface of the thighs, calves, and ankles, and mostly in women (we men get a break here). They can show up at any time, too. Occasionally they start appearing in girls as young as fifteen. What causes them? Who gets them? Why some of us and not others? (Would it make you feel better to know that an estimated 50 percent of the adult female population has this cosmetic problem?)

As you know, arteries carry oxygenated blood away from the heart to the rest of the body (oxygen in the blood keeps it red), and veins carry oxygen-depleted blood from the rest of the body to the heart (hence, the bluish red color). This exchange is going on all the time, by the way, in every little nook and cranny in your body, through miles and miles of blood vessels. (I used to know precisely how many miles, but it's been a long time since medical school.) We don't see the majority of the small veins—*venules*—because they are either microscopic or deep within the tissues.

Within each vein is a valve that, like any other valve, is there to keep the blood flowing in only one direction. As time goes on, however, for a variety of reasons, some of these valves simply give out. This may be as a result of standing too long, pregnancy, the aging process, or diminishing hormones, particularly estrogen, in women. We know for sure that the propensity for valves' wearing out or breaking down comes from our parents. In other words, heredity is probably the main factor.

When a valve within a vein breaks, blood no longer flows in one direction as it's supposed to. The result is, the vein dilates. If the vein dilates enough, and if it's close to the skin, it becomes visible to the naked eye. Hence, *spider veins.*

(Varicose veins operate on the same physiological principle, but they're bigger.) Because the small vessels are useless and meaningless (in medical lingo they're called superficial veins), they can be destroyed without compromising the circulation in any way whatsoever. On occasion a very savvy patient will ask: What if I need bypass surgery? What am I going to do if my veins are gone? Not to worry. The vessels used for bypass surgery—generally the saphenous vein, in the lower leg—lie far deeper. Those vessels that lie on the surface of the legs are really not functional. They're just bad plumbing. And in fact, when you get rid of the bad plumbing, you help the good plumbing.

Treating Spider Veins

SCLEROSING

The easiest, most effective way to treat spider veins is to inject some sort of irritating medication into them to close them down. The medical term is *sclerosing injection therapy*. The sclerosing agent that is used is either hydroxy-polyethoxy-dodecane (.25 percent to 1 percent) or sodium chloride (18 percent to 25 percent). As it is injected, the sclerosing agent pushes the blood out of the vein and causes it to collapse permanently due to irritation of the vein walls. Itching and irritation at the site may follow the injection, but this subsides quickly. Also, expect some bruising, which will slowly fade over a period of a week or two. And you may experience some temporary light brown pigment, which appears to be left behind from the leakage of blood around the vein, but this, too, will soon disappear.

Some veins require more than one injection to be eradicated safely, but once they're gone, they're gone for good. You should be aware, however, that even though the veins you get rid of are destroyed permanently, what often happens is, other little capillaries around them will dilate over time, so it may *look* as if they have reappeared. In other words, perfect legs may not stay that way, but they will definitely be very much improved. Left untended, veins just get worse with time. So after the initial cleanup, only maintenance is required. Basically I think it's well worth doing.

LASERS

When using a laser to zap a spider vein, you set the laser to be picked up by the color red. You aim at the vein, zap it with the laser beam, and the heat destroys the blood vessel. As a result, the vein shuts down permanently, and the body eventually absorbs the leftover vein tissue. Some of my colleagues prefer using the laser to sclerotherapy. Personally I don't use lasers for spider veins because, based on the lasers currently available, what I've found is that the laser has to generate too much heat to sufficiently destroy the blood vessel. Increased heat is necessary because the blood vessel under treatment is generally sizable (which is, after all, why we're treating it), and as a result, the blood is moving through it at a rapid pace. To heat traveling blood to a degree at which it will affect the surrounding vessel simply takes too much heat/energy. If you use excessive heat, you can burn the overlying skin. For just this reason, lasers now have cooling devices, but even with the cooling devices, there is still heat damage to the outer skin, which I find unacceptable. Although in most cases you can destroy the spider vein, you're going to leave marks from the burn. The marks are temporary, but "temporary" is three to six months, and no one likes to walk around with marks for such an extended period of time.

The difference between treating a sun spot and a spider vein with a laser has to do primarily with the location of the lesion. A sun spot or an age spot lies directly on top of the skin, whereas the blood vessel is inside the skin, which means you have to go through the outer layer of skin into the dermis to get to the blood vessel, requiring more heat from a laser that can easily take care of a surface sun spot.

Treating Varicose Veins

"CLOSURE"

There is a new technique for varicose veins called "closure." I do not do this procedure but it bears mentioning because some physicians use it. In this technique the physician uses a thin catheter, which contains a radio-frequency module at the tip, and threads it into a lower leg vein. The physician then manipulates the instrument up through the vein to the groin, where it rests inside the greater saphenous vein, which is the main feeding vein, or the source. It's like a river with many tributaries coming off, and you're trying to get rid of the water. You can either dam it up at different places or go to the source that's feeding the river. You close off the source, and everything below it dries up. When the tip of the catheter is safely in place (ultrasound shows the location of the tip), the physician pushes a button on the machine, and the catheter expands. As it does this, it gets little spikes, which touch the walls of the vein and transmit the radio frequency, which transmits heat. The heat causes the vein to collapse instantly. This is one way of treating varicose veins without surgery.

SCLEROSING

The treatment of varicose veins by sclerotherapy is similar to the treatment of spider veins. The difference is, when treating varicose veins, sometimes injections just don't work. It all has to do with the size of the vein. The larger the diameter of the vessel, the more blood runs through it. The greater the amount of blood, the more the sclerosing agent is diluted and therefore cannot get to the vein wall. The faster the blood is running, the less time the agent will have to work. In other words, with a larger vein, the agent we inject does not always remain in that vein long enough to do its job—that is, to irritate the vein to the degree that it closes down. Sclerotherapy works 80 percent of the time with varicose veins. With spider veins it is successful 99 percent of the time. When it doesn't work, the option of surgery, known as *vein stripping*, is always available. The current going rate for sclerotherapy in New York is from $200 to $500 a session. And you need two to six sessions to clear both legs.

CELLULITE

In the medical community, cellulite is known as *localized lipodystrophy*—a term that refers to *misshapen fat in one or several specific areas of the body*. Where does it come from?

Why do some people who are not overweight have cellulite and many who are overweight escape the problem completely? The most important question of all seems universal: *How can I get rid of cellulite?* The honest answer? Nobody knows for sure.

Here is what we do know:

- Cellulite is due to protein degeneration in the skin and its supporting structures.

- Up to 85 percent of postadolescent women have some cellulite on their bodies.

- Cellulite does not show up in women until after puberty.

- Cellulite very rarely is found on a man's body.

- Cellulite is not related to being overweight.

What exactly is cellulite? As you can see from the illustration on the next page, just below the dermis lies a thin layer of fat. This layer helps to regulate our body temperature and keeps us warm. A second, deeper layer of fat, the *scarpus fascia*, is the layer that controls the contours, bulges, and bumps in our bodies. This is the area where fat cells enlarge as we gain weight. The scarpus fascia is divided into chambers by bands of flexible connective tissue that join the lower layers of muscle to the skin. As the fibrous bands stiffen, they pull down on the surface of the skin, creating a dimpled, uneven appearance, which we call *cellulite*.

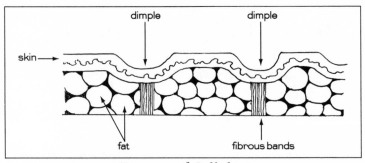

Diagram of Cellulite

Actually much of the problem has to do with metabolism. When we're very young, we generally have great metabolism, which in effect is equal to great heat conduction throughout the skin. As women age, their metabolism slows down. When the skin metabolism decreases, the skin forms a fibrous band that connects the top layer of the skin to the underlying tissues and leaves surrounding areas of fat protruding into the unbound areas. It's these bands pulling down in small areas that give the appearance of dimpling that causes cellulite, which generally shows up on the buttocks and the thighs.

To date no one knows what causes the bands to stiffen or why they do so in some and not others. For now the listed causes are aging, heredity, toxin buildup, and poor circulation. It is important to understand that no matter how stringent your diet or how much you exercise, these measures alone cannot eliminate the problem.

Treating Cellulite

Cellulite is currently treated with creams and massage—by hand or by machine. Not all these techniques are completely successful, as we shall see.

CREAMS

Cellulite responds directly to the metabolism in the area of the thighs and buttocks. When the metabolism is low, the area cools down, the blood moves slower, and the fibrous bands that lead to the dimpling of the skin form more rapidly. When metabolism is higher, the opposite occurs: the area is warmer, the blood moves faster, and there is less chance for the formation of fibrous bands. Creams with caffeine in them—and all creams for cellulite contain caffeine—stimulate the circulation because caffeine is a vasodilator: it opens the vessels. When the vessels are dilated, the blood runs faster and the area heats up, increasing metabolism. So do they work? The answer is yes, they work to stimulate circulation, but can you chemically break down the fibrous bands and get rid of the cellulite with creams? Unfortunately, no. *Once the fibrous bands have formed, they can only be broken down surgically or mechanically, by hand or by machine.*

MASSAGE

I'm partial to doing cellulite massage by hand because you can actually feel the bands break. To my mind, the cellulite machine doesn't work nearly as well, for only one reason: most operators are afraid to turn the machine up high enough because it really hurts their clients. Liposuction doesn't help either. It actually intensifies the cellulite, because the fibrous band is already pulling down on the skin, and once you take that fat below the band out, the band is going to pull down more.

Manual Massage

In Europe in the 1940s, 1950s, and 1960s, they had *cellulite masseuses.* These women would take their hands, and they would isolate the areas of your body where the cellulite was; they would take these fibrous bands between their fingers, and they would literally knead them until they broke them down physically. And that's how they still do it today. It's sometimes referred to as *manual endomologie,* which is a therapeutic massage technique that stimulates blood flow into specific areas. You have probably heard the word associated with the machine, but I am personally a purist. I prefer doing things by hand, and in my office I offer only a masseuse—the terrific Georgana.

Let's not kid ourselves. A session with one of these women hurts. And it leaves you black-and-blue. But it breaks the bands down and increases the circulation, and you'll definitely get the results you are looking for. In ten sessions, at an approximate cost of $50 each, several things happen. The bands are gone, cellulite is gone, and the skin in the whole area raises and tightens. As the sessions go on, the black-and-bluing gets less and less, and the skin develops better quality and tone. And if you do a thermogram after the cellulite massage, the massaged area is hot like the rest of the body. The process works but needs to be maintained, so after the initial run, you can expect to repeat the massages every month or so.

Mechanical Endomologie

In 1978 a physical therapist in Europe developed an *endomologie* machine, which does the same thing as the cellulite masseuse, only it does it mechanically. It sucks up the skin and rolls it and kneads it, in an effort to break the fibrous bands. The combination of suction and massage is supposed to increase blood circulation in the subdermal layers of the skin as well. I don't believe any machine is as effective as the human hands, however. And I do think most people who operate this machine are afraid to turn it up high enough, for fear of hurting the patient. So in the end the benefits are not the same, and given the choice, I'd go for Georgana, hands down. (No pun intended.)

MESOTHERAPY

Mesotherapy, which we discussed in Chapters 3 and 6, works a bit differently for cellulite. If you recall, mesotherapy involves injecting into the skin a solution of vitamins in the form of tiny droplets. The object is for the skin to act as a small reservoir so the agent you inject is released slowly over a period of three to four weeks. For cellulite we inject caffeine into the skin as mesotherapy. Caffeine dilates the blood vessels, thereby increasing the circulation, which, in turn, increases the metabolism and, finally, improves the cellulite. It works, but only to a point. The problem with doing mesotherapy for cellulite is the same as with any of the popular creams: it increases metabolism, but the fibrous bands are still there. The only way to break them up is to have someone do a cellulite massage, which breaks the bands and improves the circulation. Then, if you want, you can have mesotherapy to maintain the improved circulation.

When all is said and done, cellulite is not easy to treat. To date, there is no single treatment that's simple, accessible, and cheap that will remedy one of women's major body hang-ups. My advice is to be skeptical of the ads for products that claim to "totally, for life, rid you of those saddle-bags and that dimpled rear." There simply is not yet such a product. Perhaps in the future there will be. Until such time, though, the best you can do is get massages, exercise, eat right, and drink plenty of water.

SUN SPOTS

Sun spots, like spider veins, can spoil otherwise perfect legs. If they bother you, they can be removed and/or bleached, if you want, but bear in mind the healing period. Legs take a long time to heal. Remember, the farther away from the heart, the slower the healing.

There are numerous ways to get rid of brown spots. We can burn them off, freeze them off, peel them off, and laser them off. Again, I prefer to use a laser, for the same reasons I prefer using it on the hands: there's less abrasion than with chemical peeling, less chance to affect healthy tissue, less chance for scarring. I zap the lentigines with one power, and then I redirect the laser's intensity and just scan the legs to get rid of other tiny spots and fine blood vessels. The two-step process does several things. First, it makes your overall leg skin look better, because when you just clean up the brown spots, you're getting new skin on an older-looking "canvas." Second, it's just like shaving. You mechanically remove the outer layer of skin and send a message down to the growing layers. Third, when you heat the dermis or the growing cells, they have to go through some kind of chemical, metabolic change, and they have to go through the healing process, all of which is good. So a little bit of heat gives you cosmetic results.

TECHNIQUES FOR KEEPING YOUR LEGS IN GREAT CONDITION

Electrostimulation

Of course, I prefer good old-fashioned exercise, but if you're one of those people who absolutely refuse, electrostimulation may be the next best thing. The Slendertone machine sports wires attached to small disks. The disks are placed on specific areas of the legs, the machine is turned on, and immediately a gentle signal is transmitted through the disks to the muscle. As the strength of the signal increases, the muscle flexes exactly as it would with normal exercise. The signal then stops, leaving the muscle to relax before beginning the next stimulation. Stimulating muscles delivers additional blood flow throughout the legs. Improved circulation keeps the muscles healthy by transporting the necessary nutrients and oxygen to the muscles and by carrying away any waste products. Your legs will not only look better but will feel better as well. The general costs of these treatments are $150 per treatment.

Horse Chestnut Seed Extract

As people age, many develop *chronic venous insufficiency* in one way or another. Don't be alarmed just yet; it sounds much worse than it is. The term refers to veins' malfunctioning because the valves within them have broken down, with the result that fluid starts leaking out of the veins and into the tissues of the legs. If enough of this fluid (lymph) leaks out, it can cause *edema*, or swelling, of the legs. If a small amount of blood leaks out, you can get discoloration of the legs. When the problem worsens, the legs can become swollen, tender, and tired.

Something that really seems to help the problem is *horse chestnut seed extract*, a dietary supplement, which is FDA approved and has been around for quite a while now. Studies have shown that, by taking this dietary supplement, you can help prevent the veins from leaking; therefore, the edema goes away, the legs get smaller, the ankles get smaller, and the legs get less fatigued. The horse chestnut extract works to help stabilize the valves in the veins, making them stronger. In this way, it not only keeps veins working better, but as a result, it can also help prevent spider and varicose veins. You take two pills a day. It's equivalent to or better than wearing a pressure stocking to help reduce swelling of your legs. It starts to work in two or three weeks, with no reported side effects.

Beyond these treatments, there is currently little left to do for the legs. To keep them in premium shape, the best thing is to walk two miles a few days a week, if not more. Modern humans were made to walk, not to run—except to run away from disasters. But few of us walk. We take buses and cabs, get onto subways, climb into our cars. And then we go to the gym and believe we have to run. Think about it: the healthiest people in the world are mail carriers, because they're always walking. The healthiest exercise you can do is not running on a treadmill, it's walking two miles a day at a constant pace. It's great for your circulation and, may I add, for your psyche. Other than that, sunscreen, exfoliation, and using the bleaching agents are all excellent ways to keep your legs looking as young as you feel.

eight

Crowning Glories

Approximately half the men in the United States are affected by some sort of hair loss resulting in thinning hair or baldness. Thinning hair affects only 20 percent of postmenopausal women. But let's face it, the numbers are small comfort if you're in the wrong part of the classification. When significant hair loss happens to any of us, there is one thought, and *only* one thought, in our minds: *getting it back.*

The methods to which people have succumbed in pursuit of hair restoration—some of which are quite bizarre—are abundant enough to fill this whole book. I will spare you listing the ones I've heard of, as I'm sure you know of (or have indulged in) a few yourself. In reality, there are only two ways to replace lost hair: *medication* and *restoration.* Prescription drugs include agents that either stimulate growth or slow the inevitable. Understand that this works, but not always and not for everyone. A better way of supplanting lost hair, I think, is through restoration—that is, hair grafting. And even this treatment doesn't really restore lost hair; it merely moves it from one place to another.

MEN AND WOMEN AND HAIR LOSS

Remember the book *Men Are from Mars, Women Are from Venus?* In it the author, John Gray, addresses a myriad of issues, all of which are relevant but none of which are about hair—which is a shame, because if ever there was a *predictable* difference between the sexes, it's in the way they react to hair loss. When a twenty-five-year-old man wakes up and starts finding hair on his pillowcase, he goes crazy. But as time passes, he gets used to it and eventually may not care anymore. Or not as much. Not so for women. It's far more dramatic when a woman loses her hair. While hair loss is perfectly acceptable, if not always *desirable*, for a male, it's *never* acceptable for a female. Most of the men I see for hair loss in my practice range in age from the early twenties to the late forties. They come because either they are beginning to lose hair or they've lost it. They sit across my desk and fairly casually say, "I'm going bald. What can I do?" Most of the women who show up are usually in their fifties, and they're far more panic-stricken. The woman says: "I'm going bald. I *have* to do something!"

The *way* men and women physically lose their hair differs, too. Women start later and lose less hair overall. Whereas a male has a receding hairline in either the temple region or the crown, a woman has diffuse hair loss, creating overall thinning. Only rarely do women lose all their hair at the temples and crown. Physiologically the difference is that the female has estrogen protecting her. But once her estrogen starts diminishing, if there's also genetic programming toward hair loss (more on this in a minute), it starts kicking in.

You may be wondering, who is genetically predisposed to hair loss, and how do you know if *you* are? In other words, why do some men and women, and not others, lose their hair? It's a question I answer at least once a day.

At birth, like the rest of our characteristics, our hair has already been genetically programmed to either *be sensitive to* or *resist* certain hormones that appear in puberty. Without the genetic programming in hair follicles, the hair never falls out, no matter what. Although excessive hair loss can be caused by recent surgery, diet, medications, chemotherapy, hormones, or stress, most often, in 95 percent of cases, the culprit is heredity. In this instance the process is called *androgenic alopecia*.

But genetic programming is not all you need to lose hair. You also need conversion of the hormone testosterone (in men) or androgen (in women) to the active metabolite DHT. And the only way testosterone or androgen can be converted to that active metabolite is for you to have the enzyme that converts it. In men the enzyme that converts testosterone to DHT is *5 alpha-reductase*. Without that enzyme, there's no conversion of testosterone to DHT, and consequently, without the conversion to DHT, there's no hair loss. *You can have an abundance of testosterone or androgen, but you won't lose a single hair if you don't have the enzyme to convert them.*

And as we said earlier, if you don't have the genetic programming, you can't lose hair, no matter what. Here's the good news: if you have genetic programming and you don't have conversion of testosterone to DHT, you will not lose hair. So two things have to happen: you have to have the genetic programming, *and* you have to have the enzyme. If either is missing, you will never, to any measurable degree, lose your hair to male-pattern baldness.

The process is only slightly different for a woman. Women are protected by estrogen, which counteracts the effects of the androgen, the hormone that acts similarly to testosterone in the male and is usually responsible for hair loss in women. Even with genetic programming that predisposes to hair loss, women may be protected by virtue of having estrogen in their bloodstream. When the estrogen levels fall at menopause, that's when those destined to lose their hair will first start to see the thinning effects. So like their male counterparts, women need two things: *conversion from androgen to active metabolites* and *genetic programming*. If both factors don't exist, there can be no hair loss.

HOW HAIR GROWS

I'd like to clarify something. We've just talked about hair loss, but in fact, people don't actually lose hair. That is, it doesn't *suddenly* fall out, never to be seen again. Rather, what happens is, hair simply stops growing. Every hair on our head is genetically programmed to go through a cycle of growing and resting, growing and resting. Certain people can grow their hair down to the floor because their growing cycle is that much longer than yours or mine. Some growing

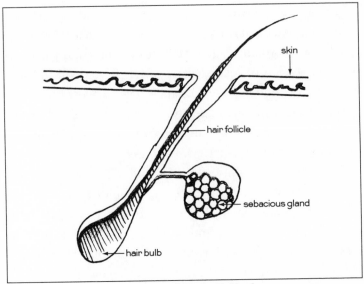

Diagram of Hair Follicle

cycles will go on for ten years before they go into the resting phase. Most hair has a growing cycle anywhere from
two to four years. It also grows only to a certain length.
When it hits that certain length, or grows for that period of
time, it goes into the resting cycle.

After a hair falls out, the follicle goes into the resting
phase for three to six months before it starts growing again.
It works on the same premise as a tulip. There's a bulb in
the ground, it puts up a flower, and the flower grows to a
certain length and for a certain amount of time. The flower
dies on top and falls off, and the leaves turn brown, but the
bulb is still there. The bulb goes into a resting cycle, usually
for a year, and then in the spring the bulb puts a new flower

up, and the flower grows for however long, the flower dies, and the cycle renews itself again.

No one with male- or female-pattern baldness goes suddenly bald, by the way. First the hair gets thinner and thinner, and eventually you find yourself among the "follically challenged." What's happening is, the hair-regeneration process is slowing down. So instead of growing for two years as nice, thick hair, it will grow for a year and then rest, then it'll grow for six months and rest, and then it stops growing altogether. The hair follicle is still there, though. Being bathed by the hormone DHT shuts it off but does not destroy it.

It was once believed that all baldness came from the mother's side, that if the maternal grandfather was bald, his grandson would be, too. That's only partially true. The balding gene *is* stronger on the mother's side; however, we're all a mixture of chromosomes and genetic DNA, so that cannot be considered a given. Take fraternal twins, for example. One can be bald and the other can have a full head of hair. We see cases in which one brother is totally bald and one has a full head of hair. So that rule is a very loose one. If your maternal grandfather is bald and your paternal grandfather is *not*, there's probably only a 60 or 70 percent chance you'll be bald. Still not great odds. If your maternal grandfather has hair and your paternal grandfather is bald, figure your chances will be around 40 percent. But if your maternal *and* paternal grandfathers are bald, be prepared.

TREATING HAIR LOSS

We said earlier that there are only two ways to treat lost hair: *Medication* and *Restoration*. Prescription drugs have come a long way in the past decade and today include products that have very good success with some people and not so much success with others. Here are the most up-to-date.

The "Baldness Pill"

Propecia is the first and only FDA-approved pill proved to treat male-pattern hair loss. We've just shown how DHT is directly related to hair loss. We also know that men with male-pattern hair loss have increased levels of DHT in the balding areas of their scalps. Propecia is designed to work directly on DHT. *Finasteride* (the active ingredient in Propecia) blocks the formation of DHT and in this way appears to interrupt a key factor in the development of inherited male-pattern hair loss. *The chemical finasteride competes with the enzyme 5 alpha-reductase for the site, so there's no conversion of testosterone to DHT.*

Sometimes I explain this by using the analogy of seats on a bus. We just saw that in order to convert from one hormone to an active metabolite hormone, you need an enzyme. The enzyme looks for a receptor site to activate it. Take seats on a bus (receptor sites). Suppose there is only one empty seat. The enzyme wants to sit there, but the drug, finasteride, gets there first and actually fits in better than the enzyme. So if finasterade is in the seat, the enzyme is blocked.

If you take finasterade, the finasterade goes in the receptor site and blocks the receptor site so the enzyme can't get in and do the conversion properly.

Proscar, the drug used effectively to treat enlarged prostate glands, is Propecia times five. With five times the level of finasteride, the drug lowers levels of the key hormone DHT, which is a major cause of prostate growth. Lowering DHT leads to shrinkage of the enlarged prostate gland in most men. (It also grows their hair back, in many cases.)

By now you may be thinking, OK, if this "baldness pill" works so well, why doesn't everyone take it? Actually a lot of people do. The reason you don't hear much about it is because people who take it don't always advertise the fact. Now understand, as far as hair goes, you won't go back to where you were when you were ten years old, but you *can* grow enough hair to cover a bald spot. This pill works better on the crown hair than on the hair in the front, but you will get a decent amount of growth in the front, too.

SIDE EFFECTS

Most medications have some sort of side effect, and this one is no exception. A certain percentage of men who take Propecia experience some kind of sexual dysfunction. About 3 percent experience either loss of libido or loss of erection. And there's always an issue about tender breasts and breast enlargement. There's another issue with this medication, a controversial one that has to do with the pill's masking prostate cancer in men. Also, the effects are not lasting. If you stop taking the drug, the side effects will resolve within weeks. Unfortunately *your results will gradually go away as well.* And here's an additional piece of important information: If

Propecia hasn't worked for you in 12 months, it is unlikely to be of benefit.

Although the FDA has not approved Propecia for women, I, like many other dermatologists, prescribe it for my female patients. The reason it has not been approved for women has to do with the active chemical—finasteride—in it. Finasteride *causes birth defects in pregnant women. Pregnant women, or women trying to become pregnant, should not go near the drug.* If the coating breaks and the insides of the pill even *touch* a pregnant woman's skin, she could possibly have a problem. The packaging alerts men: *Keep this pill away from pregnant women.* But once you're past childbearing age, which includes almost all the women who have hair loss, you can take it with no ill effects whatsoever.

Women with hair loss who take this pill have done remarkably well, better than anything else I've done for them medically. And while we have occasionally seen some extra fuzz on women's temples and on rare occasions on their cheeks and chin, they don't seem to care. They're that happy to have hair on their heads.

Minoxidil

Minoxidil, which is popularly known by its brand name Rogaine, is a vasodilator (meaning it relaxes the blood vessels), and used to be a drug prescribed for people with heart problems. The story of how it came to be a hair-restoration drug is, to my mind, one of the all-time great Horatio Alger stories. It seems back in the early seventies, there was a woman who was hospitalized for a heart attack. When her cardiologist went to see her, he noticed she had a new growth of hair on her temples, which he had not noticed before. So as a matter of course, he called his friend Gunther Kahn, a dermatologist, and asked him to see the woman. He told Kahn the patient was taking a drug called minoxidil for her heart. So Kahn went to see her, and indeed, she had temple hair, which, he decided, had to be from the minoxidil, since it was the only medication she was taking at the time. So what did Dr. Kahn do? Did he share the information with his colleagues? Did he write a scientific paper on it for the *Journal of Dermatology?* Not him. This guy was smarter than that. He *patented* it. He patented minoxidil for hair loss. *Then,* after he received the patent, he called Upjohn and said, "I recently saw a patient in the hospital who I think has grown new hair, and I'm pretty sure it's from your drug." And the Upjohn people said, "Thanks, Dr. Kahn. That's wonderful news." To which Kahn replied, "Don't thank me yet, because I also applied for the patent." The bottom line is, Upjohn ended up paying Gunther Kahn $110 million for the patent—in 1974. And that's the true genesis of minoxidil for hair loss.

WHAT MINOXIDIL CAN AND CANNOT DO

The company that manufactures minoxidil says it works well in probably 20 percent of the people who use it. It can grow some new hair—though not a lot—in the crown area. But of equal importance, it *can* slow down the hair-loss problem. The problem with minoxidil is, it comes in a liquid. In order for it to work properly, you've got to apply it four or five times a day, because of the absorption rate. There are other elements we're not entirely clear about as well. The truth is, we're not really sure *how* it works. It does some vasodilation, but it also seems to block some hormonal and some genetic properties. But again, it has a very short life in the skin, so you have to use it regularly, and few people use it as they're supposed to. Side effects include irritation and sometimes itching from the topical lotion. If you have a heart condition, you can't safely use it, because it's a vaso-dilator. The plus is, today, because it comes in a generic form, it's not nearly as expensive as it used to be. A month's supply currently costs $8 versus $150 cost of ten years ago.

Bottom line: Does it work? I've seen people using it for twenty years, and I still honestly can't say for sure. There's no test that can permit us to say, OK, Mr. Smith, Ms. Jones, here's what you look like today; here's what you'll look like in ten years if you don't use minoxidil, and here's what's going to happen if you do. I don't know what's going to hap-pen in ten years. No one does. Does minoxidil grow hair where it has already fallen out? In rare cases and even then, not totally. So far, we think it slows down hair loss. And we know for sure that it works better in women than it does in men.

Hair-Restoration Techniques

If you want to go for the quick-fix, sure-thing approach—in other words, if you want to be *positive* you'll have hair where no hair currently exists—you have three options: *scalp reduction, transplantation,* and *hair grafting.* I'll address all three types of procedures here because they are all still being done by physicians (and, unfortunately for some, by nonphysicians) across the country, but in my practice, at this time, we do only the latter. All three redistribute your own hair follicles, the roots from which your hair grows, from a place where they're in good health and growing strong to a place where there is a dearth of hair.

No matter which, if any, technique you select, for all three you should be in reasonably good health, with no conditions that would restrict elective surgery. The best candidates for surgical hair-restoration procedures are men and women with thick enough hair at the back and sides of their heads to use as the donor sites.

SCALP REDUCTION

Scalp reduction doesn't so much restore hair as it covers over the place where it no longer grows (a.k.a. the bald spot). In this procedure the doctor removes the skin from a bald area of the scalp and then, because scalp tissue is so elastic in nature, literally stretches a segment of hair-bearing skin over the scalp to cover the bald spot. Scalp reduction is frequently used in combination with hair transplantation. Since it reduces the bald area, the number of grafts required to cover the remaining areas is reduced as well.

I must admit, I have not had good success with this procedure. There may, of course, be some tricks or techniques I don't know about, but I have always had a problem with the scar. The scar always spreads eventually, and the bald area ends up coming back. This nice fine surgical line I created in the beginning was two or three inches wide five years later. I sewed the edges, I stapled them, I pinned them, and it never worked. Some doctors claim they have the answers. I don't. So I don't do it anymore.

HAIR TRANSPLANTS

I'm not going to spend a lot of time here, either, because hair transplants, as they used to be done, have become archaic. Just for the record, though, in the old days—that is to say, several years ago—we took cookie-cutter-like instruments and punched out little round circles of skin (plugs) and hair from the back of the head. We'd sew up the spots where the plugs were removed, and then we'd cut out little pieces of skin of a corresponding size in the bald area, discard them, and take the plugs from the back and put them in the front. The natural coagulation process kept the plugs from falling out, so no stitches were necessary. The plugs generally took right away. But again, the procedure is far more involved. And in part it means taking out plugs of scalp on the top of the head that may have some viable hair still growing there. My problem with hair transplantation is that it often creates a "doll-head" appearance that, to my mind, is unnatural looking. In short, it's an old technique and one that probably should not be done anymore.

HAIR GRAFTING

We do what is called *hair grafting* now. The technique differs from transplants and results in a far more natural look for both men and women. Like transplantation, it involves taking hair from a *donor site*—that is, an area that has an abundance of productive hair follicles that are not genetically programmed to fall out, generally at the back and sides of the head—and moving it to the *receptor site*, the areas where there is hair loss.

The Procedure
The Donor Site
Instead of taking lots of plugs from the back of the head, we harvest a 2- to 2½-inch-wide strip of skin, 6 to 10 inches long, depending on what is needed. Because skin is elastic, there is no problem sewing the edges together. The remaining hair, which is purposely left a bit longer in preparation for the procedure, hides the incision as it heals. The stitches stay in for ten days and then are removed. If the work is good, you should have a very fine-line scar, which no one will ever see.

Processing the Donor Hair
The strip of hair that has been removed from the donor site goes immediately to specialized technicians who, with magnifying glasses, divide it up into tiny *follicular units* with a tiny bit of skin at the base. If you magnify a picture of the hair on the scalp, what you see is that Mother Nature has placed the hair in units: units of two hairs, three hairs, four hairs. It's never just one hair here, one hair there. There actually is no pattern to these units. They occur randomly across the scalp. So that's the mission of the surgeon, then—to make sure each is placed according to nature's design.

The Receptor Site
Once the hairs have been prepared, the scalp is addressed. Three things are important at the receptor site: the area of

placement, the position of the hairs, and the angle. Actually it's a bit like gardening. You put magnifiers on, you find the bald spot, you make a tiny slit (some call this *slit grafting*) with a special tool, and you slip the new hairs and their tiny piece of skin into the slit. The skin closes immediately back over it. As for placement, it's the same gardening principle. You have a garden and you have flowers, and in between the flowers there's bare dirt. You take your spade, you make a hole, you take the flower, and you put it in the hole. That's it. Same thing with grafting. You find the bald spot, you take a follicular unit, and you plant it. We remove no skin anymore. We remove no old hairs, or hairs that are predestined to fall out or maybe not fall out. What we're doing is increasing the hair volume in the areas that are sparse, thinning, or bald.

Hair grafting is very technically oriented, very skill-oriented. In my office we do anywhere from five hundred to fifteen hundred slits on a scalp, per sitting. If you push the numbers, you lose some of the new hair because it requires a sufficient vascular supply to nourish the new hair. The more grafts you place, the more you compromise the vascular supply, and the greater chance you have of the grafts not taking. I saw one fellow who had three thousand slits, and because the vascular supply was compromised, all three thousand grafts died. And once you lose the hair, it's gone forever. So it's better, I think, to do two to five sessions and have it all take. Sessions can be spaced a month apart without any compromise to the vasculature. The procedure, which can take several hours, is not painful. A local anesthetic makes the areas temporarily numb, and afterward there is no pain at all. The beauty of this procedure is that the results should last a lifetime, because the hair you have taken is genetically programmed never to fall out.

You can have a hair-grafting procedure in the morning and go back to work that day, if you don't mind people seeing little slits or scabs. But if you have enough hair there to begin with, if your hair is thin rather than gone, you can hide them. Or there's always the ever-popular baseball cap. There are no bandages.

The risk of this, as with any surgical procedure, is always infection, scarring, and in grafting, loss of hair. But these complications are rare and, when they do occur, usually resolve quickly. Generally the hair starts to grow immediately. However, since there has been trauma to the hair in moving it, it is possible it will be thrown into a resting phase and may not start to grow until three months later, at which point it begins to grow to a good length again and thickens up. We take the stitches out in the back of the head a week or ten days after the procedure.

Caveat Emptor!

Be careful of "hair-transplant factories." Make sure you know who is doing your work. Anybody can learn the procedure of doing a hair transplant or hair grafting. And I mean *anybody!* I personally know two ex-urologists who are currently doing this procedure. The important part is, it takes judgment to place the hairs and design the hairline. *And that's an art.* It's like painting. There are good artists, and there are bad artists. It's that simple. You do good hair placement, it looks natural. How close you put the hair units, how you orient them, how you position the hairs, where you put them, and how you do it all matter. Hair can grow strangely if you place the grafts poorly or orient the hair in the wrong direction. First of all, hair grows forward, always. And because nature is random, if you try to make a neat row, it looks artificial. There's a big difference between bad work and good work. Bad work you see, and good work you don't see. And it doesn't take a trained eye to see it. So as with everything else, try to find someone who has had the procedure and, if you like it, find out where it was done. Personal recommendation from someone you know and whose hair grafting you like is always the best way to find a doctor. Of course, there's a catch-22 to finding such a person, because if the hair looks really good, you'll never be able to tell, so you won't know to ask.

Costs

The cost for grafting hair varies all across the country. It depends on you and your doctor and where it is done. In some cases the charge is by the graft—anywhere from $3 to $15 a graft. In other cases it's by the sitting, in which case it can run from $3,500 to $7,000, depending on how much work is needed. I suggest you ask up front what the overall costs will be before embarking on this procedure.

HAIR CLONING

What's really new on the horizon is hair multiplication. Hair multiplication (or cloning, for lack of a better word) addresses one of the problems that exist with grafts today, and that is, you can only remove a finite amount of skin from the back of the head before you have to stop or you'll leave a gap of skin. If you can't take a sufficient amount, you can't create a full head of hair. That's your limitation. But if you can clone your hair in a lab, you can graft as much as you need or want. And you'll get a brand-new head of hair that will last forever. Sounds good, doesn't it?

Here is how it works: The dermatologist surgically removes some hair from the back of the head. In the laboratory the little hair follicles are dissected out from the surrounding skin and placed in a special nutrient. From these minimal amounts, you can grow hundreds of thousands of hair follicles. It's just like growing skin in a dish. The physician takes these hair follicles and implants them by injection into the scalp and the hair should start growing on its own after a short while and keep growing for life. This procedure is not yet perfected, but according to several reports, it seems to be on its way.

What Can You Do to Keep Your Hair?

Get different parents. It's the *only* thing you can do. But if you think you're going to lose your hair, you can start the Propecia as early as possible. The problem is what's *really* going to happen to your hair. You can guess, based on some basic questions, but you don't really know. I'm sure someday there will be a commercial test that's predictive, but as of today there isn't one.

EXCESSIVE HAIR AND HOW TO
DEAL WITH IT: THE FLIP SIDE OF THE COIN

Mother Nature is so unfair. Just as men lose the hair on their head, they grow it in their ears; their eyebrow hair grows faster, and so does their nostril hair. A woman loses hair on her head, under her arms, on her legs, in her pubic area, and she grows hair on her chin. Women comprise the vast majority of hair-removal patients, opting most often to rid their bodies of hair on their upper lip, bikini line, legs, underarms, and around the navel. Men have unsightly hair removed from their back and shoulders, ears, and nose.

Because we address in detail the male concern about excess hair in the next chapter ("For Men Only"), and because women comprise the lion's share of hair-removal patients, this section deals mostly with excess hair on women.

Facial and Body Hair Removal

Women most often request hair removal on their upper lip, their legs, their arms, their bikini line, their chin, and lately their underarms as well as around their navel and pubic area. Many do their eyebrows, and some do their cheeks and neck as well. Facial and body hair removal can be accomplished in five ways: *waxing*, *depilation*, *epilation*, *electrolysis*, and *laser*. Of these, depilation and epilation get rid of surface hair but keep the follicle intact, and so eventually the hair grows back. Only electrolysis and laser hair removal result in the long-term or permanent reduction of hair.

DEPILATION

Depilation is the removal of hair at the skin line through shaving or by using products like Nair that dissolve the hair, which is then wiped or washed away. As the follicle is kept intact, hair begins regrowing immediately.

EPILATION

Epilation, which includes waxing and tweezing, removes hair from below the surface of the skin but leaves the follicle intact. How long this method lasts varies from person to person. However, if epilation is repeated often enough on the same area and over a prolonged period of time, the hair that grows back becomes increasingly sparse.

ELECTROLYSIS

Electrolysis involves the use of an electric needle, which is put down at the hair shaft. The technician turns on the electricity, the electric current turns to heat, and the heat destroys the hair follicle. The process can be painful and takes what seems like forever, since only one hair at a time can be treated. Also, as we discussed above, for the hair to be receptive, it must be in the "growing phase," and so hair zapped by electrolysis that is in the "resting phase" will have to be treated again. In addition there is a risk of scarring if the current is too high. So a lot of women will have pockmark holes on their upper lip and their chin, wherever. It takes a long time, because some hairs have to be treated again and again.

LASERS

Again, my favorite method of treatment. A couple of years ago, lasers came into vogue as a hair-removal technique. Lasering is a much faster technique than electrolysis and causes less discomfort, and there are very few risks, if any. As we know from previous chapters, lasers used in hair removal are geared to focus on a particular color. In hair removal the beam is calibrated to look for and home in on dark colors (the majority of hair is darker than the skin), so it passes through the lighter skin and is picked up by the dark hair root. When it hits the root, it turns it to heat and basically cooks the hair follicle. With the newer technology and newer lasers, people with dark skin and/or light hair are equally good candidates for hair removal by laser. The problem with the laser is getting enough heat to the hair follicle to destroy it without burning the skin. That can cause scarring or discoloration—which is why it's so important to have someone with great experience doing this procedure.

Permanent hair *reduction* is the only claim the FDA will currently allow for the use of lasers in controlling unwanted hair. But permanent hair reduction means that if you do the laser enough times, you eventually kill the hair follicle. This relates to the growing and resting phases of the hair. You can only destroy a hair follicle if it's active, or in the growing phase. You can aim at a follicle, but if it's at rest, nothing will affect it—not electrolysis, not lasers. And since the resting phase can last three months, in order to get all the hair at its growing phase, you have to repeat the procedure. You've got to do it until you do it in the right phase. Eventually you can kill all the hair, but it takes time.

The procedure is done on an outpatient basis. It can take from five to fifteen minutes, depending on from where the hair is being removed. You can go home immediately afterward and can return to work the next day with no problem. There may, however, be some redness for an hour or two.

VANIQA

Vaniqa is a new cream on the market that slows hair growth. We've seen already that it is necessary to have a certain enzyme for hair to grow. The chemical in Vaniqa inhibits the enzyme (but does not block it altogether), so the hair can't grow as fast. It still grows, but the growth is slowed down tremendously. Vaniqa takes six months to kick in, and as with other products for growing hair or retarding hair growth, to keep the results, you have to use it every day, forever.

nine

For Men Only

How things have changed. Only a decade ago, when men stocked their medicine cabinets, they did it with an arsenal of shaving creams, a bottle or two of cologne, a bronzer perhaps, and maybe, *maybe*, a tweezer. Today these very things fight for space with the creams and toners, bronzers and lotions, tints and moisturizers. When you walk into a cosmetic dermatologist's waiting room, do you see only women? Not anymore. Men, too, are flocking to these places in droves. And what they're seeking is just what the women want: Botox, dermabrasion, collagen, and laser treatments. This has nothing to do with men getting in touch with their "gentler" side, by the way. It actually has to do with men wanting to enhance who they already are.

Five years ago 30 percent of my patients were men. That seems like a lot, perhaps, but when you include hair care, that's not so surprising. What pleases me no end is that today the number of men I see has spiked to almost 50 percent of my practice, and half of those are seeking skin treatments. This may have to do with economic realities and all the young competition out there, but only partially. More than likely it's because men just feel great today. They work out, they have great energy, and they want to look as good as they feel.

Women do, too, of course—but in a different way and for different reasons. I may not be an expert, but from my practice I have noted universals in people's behavior, and it extends to every part of our culture. For example: Men don't mind looking a bit younger than they are, but men still don't want to look as young as women want to look. Men like keeping a few forehead lines; they like looking rugged; they almost *like* aging. Women *hate* aging. Men want to look good for their age, whereas women work diligently toward that day when people mistake their age by a decade. Men are simply more realistic about their expectations. They don't think they're going to be perfect. They don't *look* to be perfect. I have a lot of male patients in their seventies who get Botox, collagen, lasers. They've had face-lifts. But even then, they don't expect to look younger; they expect to look *better*.

Just for the record, there *is* a mild difference between men's and women's skin. Men's skin ages slower than women's because it's thicker (men have more hair follicles). In addition, most men shave their face regularly, which exfoliates it daily and causes new cells to perk up and grow. So they are ahead to begin with.

In this chapter I'll address men's cosmetic peeves. I'll tell you what solutions I use to remedy these problems, but to avoid redundancy, I will not go into detail on any of the procedures we've already discussed at length. For those—like Botox, collagen, and removal of brown spots—I suggest you look in Chapters 3 and 6, on the face and the hands.

COSMETIC PROBLEMS THAT DRIVE MEN CRAZY
Facial Furrows and Creases

If you ask a man what part of his face bothers him the most, he'll probably tell you it's his forehead and the furrows between his eyes. Laugh lines—those crinkles at the outer edge of the eyes—don't seem to bother men. I don't know why. Even when they come in for Botox, I ask if they want it as well in the laugh lines at the corners of their eyes and they say, "No, these lines give me character." (In a man it's *character;* in a woman it's *age.*) So for the forehead lines, we use Botox, and quite successfully. Men can come in on a lunch hour and return to work an hour later with no one any the wiser. Botox takes around four to six days to kick in, and then the frown lines and forehead creases are gone for up to six months. I can't say this too often, though: it takes someone who knows what he or she is doing to give Botox, because if you inject too much, you can have complications.

Brown Spots

I'm talking about *all* levels of guys, from policemen to chairmen of major corporations to teachers and doctors— they *all* come in for brown spots. They claim, "I don't want to look like my father or my mother. I don't want those *liver spots* on my face." They want to have their skin look clean—who doesn't?—and that means getting rid of all the extraneous blemishes and wrinkles.

We can chemically peel them off, but I prefer to laser them. It's easier, more direct, and I know it works very well. Lasering a brown spot leaves a purple scab in its wake, and this can last for up to a week. So I always explain that the removal of brown spots involves at least a few days' "downtime," but only if they don't want to show up at work or in public with spots. In which case they should plan their schedules accordingly.

Veins on and Around the Nose

If suddenly one day you should chance to see emerging networks of small, red or bluish lines emerging just under the skin on your face, take heed; these are not the "broken blood vessels" that most people think they are. What you're looking at are facial capillaries—also known as facial spider veins, or *telangiectasias*. Normally capillaries are so tiny, they are not visible through the skin; however, if they become abnormally enlarged, you (and everyone else) will see them. In men enlarged, visible facial capillaries (a.k.a. spider veins) appear most often around the nose and on the cheeks. While we don't yet know all the causes, it is believed that too much sun over the years, heredity, and simply the process of aging are the most common. Other culprits are lifestyle habits such as smoking and excessive caffeine or alcohol consumption. The usual suspects.

Facial spider veins can be safely and successfully removed

by laser treatment. As you know by now, lasers can be tuned to vaporize only specific colors, so a laser, in this case, would be tuned to red. The laser is directed toward the tiny vein, and it delivers precise dosages of energy to the vein with a minimal risk to the surrounding skin. The energy is absorbed by the blood vessel. The heat causes a thermocoagulation (clogging) of the blood vessel, shutting it down. Gone. The body then slowly absorbs the clogged vessel. The risk of scarring is small. If the laser is directed to red only, when you focus the laser beam on the red of a blood vessel, the blood picks up the heat from the laser, cooks (literally) the blood vessel, and destroys it. That's it. We do this for most of the fine little blood vessels in the face. Occasionally someone will come in with large blood vessels in the face, in which case we actually do sclerotherapy on the face, and it works pretty well.

Posttreatment discomfort is minimal, although there may be some swelling and redness. Perhaps some bruising will occur, but this will fade away in about two weeks. Sometimes you need multiple treatments to achieve optimal results. Darker veins take longer. Sessions are generally spaced four to six weeks apart, and after the treatment you must religiously apply sunscreen. Be aware that over time new veins may show up, but these, too, can be successfully treated.

Hair in Undesirable Places

Men hate the hair in their ears, on their backs, and in other places where it doesn't belong. Though hair removal is widely practiced and is an elective procedure that carries few risks and causes minimal pain, it is important to be realistic about the results. We know that (as discussed in Chapter 8) hair can only be killed in the growing stage. And so generally it is necessary to return to the doctor's office a few times to get the desired results. Most people successfully get rid of at least 80 percent of unwanted hair and are very happy with their new, often smoother, look. The downside is: slightly uneven skin tones can result from a laser treatment. The procedure is not cheap. It costs in the neighborhood of $1,250 for the chest, $950 for the arms, $1,250 for the buttocks, $1,000 for the shoulders and top of the back, and $3,500 for the full back. Most dermatologists will include in their fee whatever treatment is needed over the next year and in fact until the hair no longer returns.

ten

Preventions and Inventions

Prevention is everything. The first step in any skin-care routine is removing from your life the things that are doing you harm. (That is to say, smoking, tanning beds, baking in the sun, too much alcohol. But you know the list.) Understand that all aging symptoms can be, if not eliminated, at least dramatically slowed. For the first time we have a healthy sense of what works and what doesn't. The vast and diverse array of "supposed" wrinkle creams and antiaging cures is no less vast and diverse, but now we can tell which are only false promises.

We know that cosmetics companies make many products that are excellent as well as many that are a waste of money. We know that moisturizers, no matter what ballyhooed botanicals or extracts they contain, may temporarily "diminish" wrinkles but do not by any stretch of the imagination prevent them. We know that the key to any effective antiaging strategy is commitment and common sense, not over-the-counter "miracles" that may or may not materialize. But most important, we know that the single most crucial thing we can do to avert skin damage is to protect our skin, and that means *wear sunscreen, wear a hat, protect yourself against the elements when you can.* I am a fanatic about this, as you may have noticed. I know, these words have been coming at you in almost every chapter of this book. I admit it. I will sneak the message in whenever possible; that's how much I care, and that's how certain I am that it works.

Skin care is essentially about three things: protection, exfoliation, and nourishment. For the best possible skin color and texture, you want to *protect* your skin from certain elements of nature, including the sun, the wind, humidity, and certain toxins (cigarette smoke is also quite damaging). This protection comes with proper use of sunscreens and moisturizers. Next, to keep your skin healthy and as young-looking as possible, you want to exfoliate it regularly, which you can do by mechanical or chemical means. Finally, you want to *nourish* and *hydrate* it, from the outside in and from the inside out. Feeding the skin from the outside involves all the creams that contain nourishing vitamins, including vitamins A, C, and D. Nourishing it from the inside means eating right and/or taking certain vitamins and minerals, which we will discuss in depth in Chapter 12. And of course, you want to generously hydrate your skin—both by drinking lots of water and by locking in moisture.

PROTECTION

What is the best of all possible ways to *protect* your skin? Here I go again. Sunscreens and moisturizers are critical. But probably sunscreen is more important. Let's face it, if you're going to go out in the sun, you're going to age your skin. So I'd say sunscreen should head the list of preventions—and the higher the SPF, the better.

Sunscreens

What exactly *is* sunscreen, and what is meant by SPF? Chemical sun protection—a.k.a. *sunscreen*—works in two ways. First, it contains titanium dioxide, a chemical that literally reflects the sun's rays away from your skin, and second, it absorbs the sun's rays and neutralizes them. Basically, an SPF (sun protection factor) is calculated as the time a person can stay in the sun without burning. For example, if you lie out on a beach—let's make it a Hawaiian beach while we're at it—unprotected for fifteen minutes and then you begin to burn, fifteen minutes is your minimal *erythema* dose. So we know you burn after fifteen unprotected minutes. Now let's start all over and put a sunscreen on. You go out into the sun, and you don't burn until an hour has passed. That means it takes you four times as long to burn, so the SPF of the sunscreen is 4. In other words, you can stay in the sun four times as long without getting sunburned. With an SPF of 8, you can stay in the sun twice as long as with an SPF of 4, or two hours, without getting burned. That's how the numbers are determined.

But here's the first problem: not everyone's skin is the same; some people will burn before fifteen minutes and some after thirty. So "fifteen minutes" is an arbitrary time frame. Here's something else. Usually, when the SPF is determined for any particular sunscreen, the testing is done in the lab on skin in just the right condition, exposed to the perfect humidity, in the perfect environment. The subject doesn't move or sweat. The perfect amount of cream is put on, the perfect amount of time is waited until the cream becomes activated, and then the test is done.

Well, who does *that*? No one!

Which is why you probably should use the highest level of protection you can find. My thinking on this has changed over the last five years. Originally I thought it didn't matter if you used an SPF 15 sunscreen or an SPF 30 sunscreen. Then, when I realized that people are human and no one is going to pay attention to the "sunscreen rules," I came to the conclusion that you might as well start with the highest number you can, and get the most protection you can, so at least you have a head start. Again, technically, in the lab, if you use an SPF 15 correctly, you're perfect. But that's not life.

Did you know that when you put sunscreen on—any chemical sunscreen—it takes *at least a half hour* for the chemical to go through the skin and become activated? It's true. That message, by the way, is on every sunscreen or sun protection you buy. It's on the back of the package. Of course, no one ever reads the directions, and no one ever *follows* them. I have a very good friend who is connected to the cosmetics industry in a big way and has been most of his life. He is also my patient. He has very badly sun-damaged skin, and he has a big problem even using sunscreen because it irritates his skin. I casually said to him one day, "I know you know to put the sunscreen on half an hour before you go out in the sun." And he asked, "Why would I do that?" "Hey," I said, "it's a chemical! Remember? It has to interact with the proteins in your skin to become effective." He said, "I didn't know that." I told him it is on every label on every single bottle or tube of sunscreen, to which he replied, "Labels? I never read labels." I said to him, "How can you be a top level executive of a major skin-care company and not read your own labels?" He was really embarrassed and said he would, but if I know my friend, he probably still has people reading them for him.

So now you, like my buddy, have been forewarned: if you wait until you get onto the beach to protect yourself, that first half hour you're out in the sun, guess what? Your protection is *zero*. You are, essentially, "sun-naked."

And here's the second problem: when you're at the beach putting on your first coat of sunscreen, you're sweating, you're moving around, you're not putting the right amount on, you're putting it on skin that's no longer really dry, you have your bathing suit in the way, you're touching, you're moving, you're dancing, you go in the water. Good-bye protection. Gone. And as if that weren't enough, as the sunscreen absorbs sun, the chemical is neutralized and loses its potency. Eventually you need a fresh supply, which is why you're supposed to reapply a new layer every two hours. How many people do you know who do *that*?

There are many myths about the sun, the skin, and sunscreen, so while we're on the subject, let's just set the record straight.

- *Myth 1: Only fair-skinned people need sunscreen.* Wrong. Wrong. Wrong. Every skin type and color—fair, olive, dark—needs sunscreen. The sun is color-blind.

- *Myth 2: You need to buy a different sunscreen for the face than for the body.* Not true. That's purely a Madison Avenue marketing thing. Sunscreen marketed for the face can certainly be used on the body and vice versa.

- *Myth 3: You are only protected if you specifically use a "sunscreen" product.* Not true. For everyday wear, you don't need to use a "sunscreen" product. If you buy a moisturizer with sun protection factor, it's the same thing as buying a sunscreen. It's the active chemical that protects you, not the base. Any moisturizer—and people prefer moisturizer to sunscreens because they're lighter and not as greasy—will give you the same protection, as long as it contains an SPF 15 or better sunscreen. An SPF 15 sunscreen is identical to a 15 SPF in moisturizer. The sun-care companies, with a boost from Madison Avenue, have hoodwinked us into believing that if you're not wearing a sunscreen, you're not really getting sun protection. But again, it doesn't matter. A 15 is a 15 is a 15, whether it's in water, cream, moisturizer, or tomato juice. The base is irrelevant, except for how it feels to you.

- *Myth 4: I'm tan, so I'm protected from the burning rays of the sun.* Not true. The best tan in the world is equal to an SPF of 4.

- *Myth 5: If you want a great tan, tanning parlors are better for you than the rays of the sun.* Absolutely, positively untrue! Dermatologists love tanning parlors. Why? They're great for our business! They create more skin cancers and more wrinkles than anything does. And incidentally going to a tanning parlor is exactly like going to the beach. The skin damage you inflict upon yourself—and *pay* for, no less—is cumulative.

Now, on the other hand, *self-tanners* are terrific. They're just vegetable dyes, which, when they interact with the outer layer of the skin, deliver a tan/orange color. How they work for you, personally, depends on several factors. The chemistry of your skin and the formulation of the product are key. The chemical interaction of the tanner with the proteins of your skin will be unique to you, so whereas I may use Esteé Lauder and look great, you may find it turns your skin orange. So you need to experiment to find a self-tanner that works for you. Also, it depends on *how* you use the product. You must first "degrease" your skin, because you need the protein interaction with the chemical to give you the coloration. If you put a self-tanner on oily skin, it's not going to come out the right color, and it may look streaked or blotchy, depending on the oily spots. If your skin is oily, you want to use an astringent or witch hazel first. Then apply the tanner, and wash your hands afterward or you'll have orange hands for days. If you've never tried a self-tanner, I suggest you do so. It's worth it, believe me. I use it all the time.

Moving off the beach and back into the real world, the hard-and-fast rule is: *everyone should wear sunscreen 365 days a year*. Here's why: When it comes to sun, the skin is like a sponge. You absorb a little sun, the skin keeps it; absorb a little bit more, it adds to what you've already got. It's cumulative. So today if you're outside without sunscreen, on a nice, sunny, cold day, the fifteen minutes you're outside walking about, even in the snow—*especially* in the snow (which reflects the sun in a big way)—that fifteen minutes of sun is absorbed by the skin and captured. *For life*. Eventually a patch of skin that's been saturated with sun absorption or radiation breaks down and leaves in its wake a brown spot, a broken blood vessel, a pre–skin cancer, or a skin cancer.

UV (ultraviolet) blocking eyeshadow and lipstick are important, too, if you can find good ones. They're important for lips, mostly, because the lips don't have that extra stratum corneum layer to protect them. Lips are highly sunsensitive. If you get a skin cancer on the lip, it's very bad news. The UV lip protectors can be found at your local drugstore or department store, and they're not expensive, so there's no excuse not to use them.

Moisturizers and Hydration

MOISTURIZERS

Moisturizers work in two ways: by *delivering water to the skin* and by *locking in water that's already there*. In one form or another, *all* moisturizers contain chemicals or ingredients known as *humectants* that suck water from the environment and deliver it into the skin. They all do it. In other words, with today's technology, moisturizer, essentially, is moisturizer. Which then leads into the question: What is the difference between moisturizers from CVS and moisturizers from Christian Dior?

My answer? *The way their names are spelled* (and the cost, of course). That's it.

Well, OK, I'll admit that there are some very slight differences here and there. For example, there are water-based moisturizers, cream-based moisturizers, and oil/water-based moisturizers. Some moisturizers may seal in the water better than others do. The greasier they are, the better they lock in the moisture. But the greasier they are, the less capable they are of bringing in the moisture from the environment to the dermis.

Here is a major pet peeve of mine. I have just said that moisturizer, in effect, is moisturizer. Ditto for eye creams and face creams. Most moisturizers contain humectants, exfoliants, and vitamins. But no one ever tells you how much of each is in the jar or tube. That is because *the manufacturers don't have to!* When it comes to alpha or beta hydroxies, for example, very few, if any, cosmetics companies label their bottles or jars with the percentages of active ingredients contained therein, so you have no way of knowing what you're buying. They can say they contain alpha hydroxy or vitamin C (which is listed on labels as L-ascorbic acid) or vitamin A. In truth, one drop is all they need to legitimately make the claim.

For the purposes of this book, I did a minisurvey, which involved asking various representatives from cosmetics companies why they did not include the percentages of

AHAs or BHAs on the labels of their products. One told me that to do so would reveal the cream's "recipe." What would stop you, she asked, from copying our formula, for which we paid a fortune in research costs? Well, let me tell you, that makes *no* sense, because all the ingredients are listed on the package, and any chemist can break down the cream and find out the percentages in a minute. The ingredients have to, by law, be listed in order of percentage, with the greatest percentages listed first and the least, last. Smart companies simply separate the ingredients into active and inactive, so there are two sections on the label. They can say, for example, "active ingredients: alpha hydroxy and glycolic acid," but instead of putting them low on the list, they separate them out.

I asked the same question of a cosmetic company representative behind the counter at Bloomingdale's. She told me the reason no percentages were listed was to prevent a "drug war." I quote: "If we put in 5 percent, what's to stop the next company from putting in 6 percent? Which would you spend your $65 on?"

My theory is far more practical. I think the reason they don't tell us is because they choose to include in the formula the bare minimum of any active ingredient. That is simply because anything of measurable strength might cause a facial irritation. If you get a facial irritation, what do you do? You switch brands. And there goes not only the face cream but the lipstick and the mascara sales as well. Cosmetics and skincare products should be regulated as food is. Their manufacturers should be required to list on the label the precise percentages of the key ingredients. *All* key ingredients.

You can do your own mini—research study the next time

you're in your local drugstore. Look around for the Keri lotion, Lubriderm, Cetaphil, Eucerine, and Aquaphor. Seek out Nivea's new Visage cream with CoQ10, or Neutrogena Healthy Skin. Examine the labels. You will see that some contain SPFs, some AHAs, some BHAs. Test them. Some feel drier, some greasier; some feel slippery, and some are tinted. Some are for oily skin and some for dry. Bottom line? They are all pretty much identical.

Now go to the makeup aisles of Saks or Bloomingdale's or Henri Bendel. There you will find Chanel, Borghese, Lazlo, Clarins, and Lancôme. And the ubiquitous La Mer. La Mer, manufacturer of high-priced products sold in the better spas and shops, puts plant extract into its moisturizers and creams. The plant extract is a special humectant, for which you are paying a fortune, that *still* works only to bring water from the outside into the skin. *There is no magic in moisturizer.* They all do the same thing as Lubriderm.

Estée Lauder, for example, advertises hyaluronic acid (which, incidentally, comes from rooster combs) in a product called "Night Repair." Restylane, the material we inject for wrinkles, is hyaluronic acid gel. Hyaluronic acid has a very important role in the skin's basic moisturization and hydration. It is an excellent humectant, meaning it sucks water into the skin and seals in the water. It is also a natural ingredient of the dermis of the skin. Night Repair ads say that hyaluronic acid goes through the outer layer of the skin and into the dermis. But hyaluronic acid is already in the skin naturally. It's the substance in the foundation of the dermis that holds lots of water.

And by the way, it doesn't matter if you put lima bean

extract (as found in Clarins Hydra-Balance Serum) or cran-
berries into your creams. Ninety-nine percent of those addi-
tives do not go through the top barrier of the skin. Very
little topical vitamin C goes through the skin. Very little
topical vitamin A goes through the skin. All these fancy
extracts sound exotic, but most of them do not go through
the skin.

*As soon as an ingredient goes through the skin, the product is no
longer a cosmetic but a drug.* By definition of the FDA, a cosmetic is a cream or lotion that, when applied to the external
surface of the skin, beautifies the look of the skin. A drug is
an agent that goes through the skin and changes something
physiologically or chemically or changes the anatomy of
the skin.

The alpha and beta hydroxies, which actually *do* affect the
anatomy and the physiology and the chemistry of the skin,
ushered in a whole gray area called *cosmeticeuticals.* A cos-
meticeutical is a cosmetic that does contain some properties
that change the skin's anatomy. It's a word you'll be hearing
increasingly as cosmetics become more high-tech.

Caveat Emptor!

*When you see ads that say, "Wrinkles reduced by 42 percent," be
sure you understand what that really means.* If I dry my skin
out, and then I put on moisturizer, I reduce wrinkles by 42
percent. Plain old water will do the same thing. It hydrates
the skin. When you put your fingers in the water for an
extended period, what happens to them? They plump up.
Water hydrates skin. End of story.

When I was a resident working in the emergency room, if

a patient came into the ER unconscious and we wanted to know whether he was dehydrated, we took his chest skin and pulled on it ever so slightly. When skin is hydrated, it has many elastic properties. It bounces back. When skin lacks water, an area that's been pulled up sits there like a little tent and goes down slowly. You can spot dehydration by that simple maneuver. The best way to hydrate the skin is internally. But if you want to lock moisture in or add it, that's great, too.

Can you do it with L'Oréal Plénitude or Lancôme Absolue? Sure. They're both great. But neither of them is any better than Keri lotion. If it makes you happy to spend the extra money—and you're not alone, believe me—then why not? The cosmetics industry thanks you.

How else can you hydrate your skin? Water. Water may just be the world's best-kept beauty secret. Our bodies are made up of more than 50 percent water. We lose about three quarts each day, through the natural acts of urination, respiration, and perspiration. Water flushes out waste materials and benefits the skin by acting as an internal moisturizer. It is recommended (of course, you know this already) that you drink at least eight glasses of water—clear, fresh, tap or bottled water will do just fine. However, make it water—not coffee, tea, or soda. Plain, unadulterated water. You can never drink too much.

And while we're on the subject, what you *can* drink too much of is alcohol. In the realm of skin care, alcohol causes dehydration, which deprives your complexion of the moisture it needs to stay soft, smooth, and youthful. Alcohol in excess overtaxes the liver, which is the organ that helps keep impurities from reaching and harming other systems in your body. Alcohol consumption can lead to broken or distended capillaries, especially over the nose and cheeks. To maintain a clear complexion, it's a good idea to consume alcoholic beverages in moderation.

Finally there's the bath. It's far more effective than you may know. Have you ever sat too long in the bathtub? Remember what happens to your hands? They turn white and look like prunes. What do you think that is? Most people will answer that the water has dried out the skin, but in fact it's just the reverse. The water takes out the *oils*, and all that "pruney" appearance is water absorption *into* the skin. The pruney look is just accentuated ridges in the skin, similar to what happens if you drop a cube of bread into a glass of water. It blows up, and the edges become more prominent. We think we've dried ourselves out when we've actually hydrated ourselves to death.

The problem with soaking too long is that the evaporation process that follows is brutal. What happens is, you come out of the bath, and the evaporation process makes the pruney look disappear very quickly. But as the water on your skin is sucked into the air, so are more of the oils and even more of the water that's in your skin. It's like licking your lips. As soon as you do, they get even drier. Same principle. Add moisture to skin, and as it evaporates, it takes extra moisture from your skin with it. Gone. Faded into the atmosphere. So the next time you come out of the tub with pruney hands, you should apply Vaseline to lock the moisture in.

Of course, you can always add water to your environment. Humidifiers can replenish the moisture in your home or office. They are not that expensive, and the difference, especially in the winter, will be remarkable.

EXFOLIATION

As the skin ages, the stratum corneum, which is the top layer of the epidermis, doesn't lock in water as well as it did, and as a result, a lot more water from your skin continually escapes into the atmosphere. In young skin the cells in the stratum corneum and the epidermis exist in a more organized fashion, which locks the water in. Exfoliating the skin reorganizes the cells in the outer layer so that you have less water lost through the skin. It's also helpful in other ways.

Back in Chapter 1 we showed how the skin is always growing and always exfoliating. Your skin probably turns over every fourteen to twenty-one days when you're young. As you get older, the skin renews itself less often, and the top layer becomes disorganized. When this happens, dead skin, instead of working its way through the stratum corneum and being shed microscopically, gets trapped in the pores. The result is a little ball of skin that can't go anywhere. We call these *millia*. Some people call them whiteheads, but they're really not whiteheads or acne. Also, as the skin loses elasticity, the pores shrink down and start holding on to oil, which eventually oxidizes and produces blackheads. Think of a pore as a round circle being pulled out by elastic bands. The elastic bands keep the pore open and allow the oil to flow. Break the elastic bands and the pore shrinks and holds on to the oil. You can remove blackheads, of course, but they only fill up again. If you fix the elasticity of the skin either by lasering it or chemically, the problem goes away.

Alpha and beta hydroxies are both great and can do an excellent job of exfoliating the skin, which is what we use them for. The problem with using alpha hydroxy acids, and now including beta hydroxy, is that you never know the percentage of AHAs or BHAs in the cream on which you're spending your money. In the world of over-the-counter cosmetics today, products can contain as little as .1 percent of an ingredient and still claim that ingredient on their labels. Most over-the-counter alpha hydroxies contain very little alpha hydroxy. That's because, as noted earlier, the company gets worried about the customer's developing red and irritated skin and not wanting to use the product anymore. The company will then lose that customer not just for the alpha hydroxies but for the eye shadow, the makeup, the mascara, everything. So they're all very careful not to put a lot of that chemical in their products.

The products you get from your physician can have as high as 20 or 30 percent AHAs or 2 percent BHAs. The higher the percentage you can tolerate, the better it works. Continual exfoliation, whether it's chemical or physical, keeps the skin looking and behaving younger. Alpha hydroxy has four different types: *glycolic* acid, *lactic* acid, *malic* acid, and *pyruvic* acid. There's only one beta hydroxy, and that's *salicylic* or alphasalicylic acid. By the way, using lactic acid for exfoliation has been around since Cleopatra. Remember how Cleopatra used to bathe in sour milk before meeting Mark

Antony? Apparently she knew long before we did of its remarkable exfoliating properties.

If you have dry skin, should you avoid AHAs? The answer is no, because when you exfoliate the skin, you're making the outer layer, the stratum corneum, younger. When it's younger, it locks in the water better. And that, as we've just seen, is the object. But there's an extreme. In other words, you've got to find an AHA that exfoliates the skin without causing irritation. That's the trick, because 4 percent may be great for you, and 8 percent may be great for me, and someone else may do well at 2 percent. It all depends on your skin's tolerance to it. You want to use it so your skin just gently flakes at first and then gets used to it.

NOURISHMENT

Creams, lotions, and ointments nourish our skin from the outside in. To nourish from the inside out takes vitamins, minerals, and the like, which we will discuss in detail in Chapter 12.

Cleansers

This is actually the first step in the nourishment process, because the cleaner the facade, the more easily your lotions and creams will be absorbed. Everybody has combination skin. We all have oily zones and we all have dry zones, and basically you should find a cleanser that works for the driest

part of your skin and then address the oily part with anything that takes the oil away. There are some people who
will tell you that if you take the oil away too much, the oil
glands just fight back and produce more oil. Also, as little
oil glands in the skin produce less oil, they grow in size trying to make up for it. So stripping your skin of oil is not the
answer. If you think you're oily and you go out and strip it
off, it'll just make more oil. You need to find a cleanser that
will reduce your oil. Those little pads that have powder on
them are best. The thing is, as you get older, the glands are
going to stop working so hard. When the oil glands shrink,
your skin gets wrinkled. So be happy if your skin is a little
oilier. If the oil glands get physically larger and become
unsightly bumps, they are sebaceous hyperplasias; electro-
destruction or laser therapy can remove these.

What you should look for in a cleanser is one that doesn't
rob the skin of its natural oils. You can use a product like
Cetaphil, which is a nonlipid cleanser, and it's a liquid. The
problem is, people psychologically don't like to use liquid
cleansers. They like bars. But it's hard to make a bar that is
as gentle as a liquid cleanser. If you must use a nonliquid
cleanser, Dove and Camay are both excellent, and now
Cetaphil comes in bars, too.

*What's the truth about going without makeup periodically to let
your skin breathe?* First of all, skin doesn't. You breathe with
your lungs. Second, today it's hard to buy bad makeup. In
today's world of cosmetic formulation, there is no reason to
forgo makeup, if you like it. Makeup doesn't clog the pores
anymore, either. Years ago makeup was so thick that pores

couldn't clean themselves, and they'd get clogged, resulting in breakouts. But formulations today literally sit *around* the pore, so makeup, essentially, is just fine.

Lotions, Creams, and Ointments

Which creams are the best? Actually there are lotions, creams, and ointments. A lotion is mostly water, a cream contains more oil, and an ointment is almost pure oil. People have misconceptions about what works best. And of course, there are social differences. Americans don't like anything greasy. Europeans *only* like greasy face products. Europeans hate lotions, because they're not thick enough. They are more comfortable with the greasy feeling. Americans go for the lighter, the better in most cases. There are pros and cons to all. Basically if you have water as your first component in the lotion, the water gets sucked into the skin better and actually hydrates the skin better. But it doesn't provide as much of a protective barrier for locking in the water, so ointments are better in that regard.

The trick is to find a formulation that has enough water and enough locking-in quality. It's a very hard formulation to do, though. There isn't really a product that does it well today. It's almost like trying to put night and day together.

Should you buy into the "night cream"/"day cream" advertising blitz? Not really. There is actually no measurable difference between night creams and day creams. One may be a bit thicker, but it just means there's more oil in it. I think most of it is a Madison Avenue ploy to get the customer to buy more than one cream for her dressing table. There was a company in Europe that sold 122 different moisturizers. It had a cream for the nipple, a cream for the breast, a cream for under the breast; a cream for the upper arm, a cream for the lower arm, a cream for the hand, for the fingers, for the nails, and for the cuticles. You get the point. Sound smart? The customers were smarter. I think the company went out of business. It's just not necessary to have all these. To paraphrase Gertrude Stein, a cream is a cream is a cream. Enough said.

Vitamin C creams contain antioxidants, which stimulate collagen and fight free radicals that cause skin aging. Look for pure vitamin C, which is listed as L-ascorbic acid. Do these work? It all depends on your skin and how much vitamin C penetrates your skin. It never penetrates 100 percent. But it helps.

SPAS

Because this chapter is called "Preventions and Inventions," I'd like to add a word of caution about spas in the hope that I may just prevent you from making a major skin-care mistake.

Spas are so generic today; I don't know what a spa is anymore. I don't think *anybody* knows what a spa is. Spas have evolved to such a degree that many of them seem to be in the medical business as well as the beauty business. Many spas, at least in New York City, now have physicians associated with them but not exactly on the staff or present in the physical plant. To me this raises many questions: Does the doctor bring in the spa business, or does the spa bring in the medical business? Who dictates who does what? Who is in charge? How is it all orchestrated? Also, in New York, aestheticians can legally do most of the procedures previously outlined in this book. As a physician, I am concerned. My suggestion is: before submitting to any cosmetic procedure in a spa or by an aesthetician, make sure you know who is doing it and what his or her background is. In Chapter 14 I discuss how to find a good cosmetic dermatologist. I suggest you read that chapter and consider your options before submitting to any procedures on your face in a spa.

eleven

Smiles, Glorious Smiles

We have just seen all the wonders that can be worked to solve the problems natural aging brings to the skin. So just when we think we have the "age thing" licked, we find life has also taken its toll on our smiles. There's no way around it. Just from everyday living, our teeth become discolored—though it's true some of us are affected worse than others. Still, a close look in the mirror will probably reflect teeth that have darkened from smoking, coffee, drinking wine, and even eating that most wonderful of all antioxidants—blueberries! What's worse, from years of normal wear, teeth get shorter, they chip, and they become crowded or crooked from natural changes in the underlying, supporting bone structure. I need not go on. You get the picture.

But fortunately you do not have to *accept* the picture.

You can change so much in your mouth. It is as easy as a visit to your favorite dentist. Today a small amount of dental contouring can make a huge difference in the way you feel about the way you look. Years ago the only process available to whiten teeth, repair unsightly gaps, or straighten out uneven, chipped, and broken teeth was to disguise the problem with a cap or crown. That involved shaving a tooth down to a peg, which meant removing a lot of healthy tissue, sometimes resulting in a weakened tooth structure. It also could mean an unnaturally thicker or bulkier tooth, which, because of primitive materials, stood glaringly out in the crowd. Today there are a myriad of options—all of them affordable (although some, admittedly, more so than others) and all certainly efficacious—to address these or any problems with your smile that might be bothering you. Welcome to the high-tech world of aesthetic dentistry.

Caveat Emptor!

Just because your dentist keeps your teeth healthy does not necessarily mean he or she produces equally good aesthetic results. Check out the person you want to use. Look at before and after photos. Better yet, look at the work directly, if possible. When all is said and done, *the object*, as we have repeatedly said throughout this book, *is to look like you, only better.* And that means you must look natural. Bottom line? You don't want people wondering what you did to yourself. You just want a beautiful, natural smile.

Currently four doorways can lead you there: bonding, porcelain laminates, bleaching or whitening, and what Dr. Larry Rosenthal, an aesthetic dentist in New York City, calls "smile design."

BONDING

Along the evolutionary axis of modern dentistry, the precursor to bonding—composite fillings—arrived on the scene around the mid-1960s, bringing with it the advent of aesthetic dentistry. These "tooth-colored fillings" could be closely matched to your teeth and were used to repair decay in the front teeth. Before that time the only kind of fillings available to restore decayed teeth consisted of amalgam (silver) or gold for back teeth and silicates for small areas in the front. While these metal fillings worked well, they could also be highly perceptible. Once the silver had been in any tooth for a while, it darkened, giving the entire tooth a dark appearance. Gold inlays, the "better filling," while wonderfully sturdy and long-lasting, still caught the eye like a flashbulb with every spirited laugh.

The new, "vanishing" tooth-colored fillings were made of a plastic dental resin composed of microscopic filler particles. Because the composite was not strong enough to withstand the chewing pressure of the molars, it could only be used in the front teeth. Soon the material was strengthened to the point where it could safely be employed throughout the mouth with excellent results. Today these fillings can be matched perfectly to any tooth color and made with the same degree of translucence, both of which allow the fillings to blend in imperceptibly with the rest of the teeth.

The decade of the 1980s brought even better news for smile aficionados with the advent of a new process called *bonding*. Dentists bonded teeth by cementing a tooth-colored resin to the existing teeth in order to change their shape, color, or size or to repair defects. Done well, composite bonding can close small gaps between front teeth, repair small chips and cracks, conceal discoloration, and even protect areas of tooth exposed by gum recession. And fortunately tooth bonding requires only the smallest change, if any at all, to the original tooth.

The Process

First, the composite is compounded to mimic the color and translucency of your tooth. Next, the tooth is prepared by gently abrading the area to be repaired by brushing on a mild acid gel, which barely etches the surface. The composite is generally applied in several layers in order to duplicate the depth of color that occurs in a natural tooth. A high-intensity curing light is passed over the repaired area several times to set the bonding. Finally, the tooth is polished to a beautiful shine. The procedure is virtually painless and often requires no anesthetic.

How long bonding lasts depends on many factors. For some the bonded tooth will look as good fifteen years later as it did the day it was done. On rare occasions, though, you can get staining on the margins of the bonding after one or two years, and you may require some touch-up work. An advantage is that it can be touched up or replaced easily. The average life expectancy of a bonding is five years. The price is approximately $250–$500 per tooth.

PORCELAIN VENEERS

Porcelain veneers followed bonding by about ten years. This process, which was developed in the mid-1980s, resulted from the development of special materials that allowed dentists to bond to a tooth a fitted wafer of porcelain half a millimeter thick—the thickness of a newborn baby's fingernail—and have it permanently stick to the tooth beneath, despite all kinds of pressures and saliva and solutions and temperature changes. In fact, some of the technology for the bonding process came straight from space, or at least from the National Aeronautics and Space Administration program. Back in the late 1970s, NASA was faced with the problem of protecting the exterior of its spaceships as they sailed into the heavens through numerous temperature and atmospheric changes. The requirement was for a material that was highly durable yet light in weight. Ceramic tiles met both of the requirements and in addition were able to withstand drastically changing temperatures. Why? Because ceramics don't conduct thermal changes. This becomes clear if you stand barefoot on the tile surround of a swimming pool. In the winter you will notice that the tiles are cool, not cold like the outside temperature. And if you stand there in the summertime, they are still cool.

Taking their cue from NASA, dentists began using porcelain as an exclusive material in the mouth for many of the same reasons. Porcelain veneers keep an even temperature, despite what you eat or drink. They maintain their integrity and shape, and they stay smooth and highly polished.

Porcelain laminates allow for more precision in contouring

the teeth than does bonding. Moreover, they are a superior restoration material for the teeth all around. Physically, veneers strengthen aging teeth that have begun to fracture. Cosmetically, veneers can be shaped to build up teeth and thereby fill in the shadowy corners of the mouth, which dentists call *negative space*. Positive space is when you see white, as in the teeth themselves. If there are too many teeth, or the teeth are too bulky, that's too positive. Too small or too short teeth create negative space. The dentist can be minimally invasive and still change the shape of a tooth, the size of a tooth, the length of a tooth, close a space between the teeth, and even widen smiles by widening the teeth or the dental arch ever so slightly. More good features: veneers are highly resistant to wear, which make them very long-lasting. They rarely discolor, even after many years. And in the hands of an excellent cosmetic dentist, you are going to look ten years younger, immediately. A wonderful benefit of porcelain is the immediate gratification it brings while at the same time requiring no surgery, no stitches, no pain, and no recovery time.

The Process

Porcelain laminates can be done in as few as two major visits of two to three hours each plus two shorter postop visits to check the temporary work. These visits can be scheduled anywhere from a few days to two weeks apart. The procedure begins with an initial consultation, at which you may be able to view your current and future smiles via computer imaging in beautiful Technicolor and Cinema-Scope. In planning the overall results, the dentist will take into consideration several factors that affect the outcome. These include the shape of your face, your skin color, the shape of your lips, and your tooth color. Also factored in will be the original color of your teeth, because while it is true that whiter teeth are synonymous with youth, going *too* light, while tempting, may look artificial, which would be the absolute antithesis of the natural smile effect you're trying to achieve. The size of your teeth is also important. Again, longer teeth are synonymous with youth, as teeth shorten after years of wear and tear.

After your consultation, the dentist takes impressions of your teeth, and a cast model is constructed. The veneers are built on this model. Some dentists prefer that you have eight to ten teeth covered on the top and, if you choose to do the bottom as well, then another eight to ten there, too. The number of teeth covered depends on how many of your teeth are visible when you smile. The object is to make you look as natural as possible.

You will leave the dentist's office and will be scheduled to return when your porcelain veneers are ready. When you come back for the second visit, the veneers are placed over your teeth temporarily and adjustments made. Finally they are bonded with a laser or plasma arc light to the surface of the teeth. When the veneers are in place, the teeth are polished, and you are on your way.

Prices for this procedure vary across the country, with a base of around $1,000 per tooth, give or take several hundred dollars, depending on what you need and who does the work. Overall, time in the dentist's chair runs from six to eight hours.

TOOTH BRIGHTENING

The 1990s was the decade of "white teeth." That is when commercial tooth bleaching was introduced in America, and it seems the whole population became enthralled with the idea of having a whiter smile. The charge was led by a generation of aging baby boomers seeking to recapture the youthful appearance they possessed before years of wine and cigarettes took their toll. Today, boomers notwithstanding, tooth bleaching is the most requested form of cosmetic dentistry. Fortunately it is widely available to everyone, including you.

Of course, in the end you still may not be mistaken for Julia or Brad, but your smile can certainly light up a room as theirs does. *If* you are a good candidate for this process, that is. Actually everyone is a candidate for tooth bleaching, but the results will be somewhat worse in certain populations than in others. For example, teeth that are grayer, rather than brown, are more difficult to bleach. Also, teeth exposed in utero or in childhood to tetracycline are extremely difficult to lighten. Bleaching is not recommended for people with severe gum disease or bleeding, cracks in the teeth, or cavities. Nor is it for women who are pregnant or nursing. If you have very sensitive teeth, periodontal disease, or teeth with worn enamel, your dentist may discourage bleaching.

As the name implies, tooth bleaching—or tooth whitening, as it is often called—is a process of lightening the color of teeth. It is used to erase stains that come from years of coffee, tea, red wine, and cigarette smoke. And it will lighten teeth that have darkened because of age or are naturally yellow or dark.

The Process

There are four tooth-bleaching methods from which to choose, each involving varying degrees of effectiveness and cost:

- *Dentist in-office power bleaching:* The dentist coats the teeth with a strong hydrogen peroxide gel and beams an argon laser or plasma arc light on them to activate the process. It takes an hour and can leave your teeth eight to ten shades lighter. It lasts two years or more, depending on the care you take afterward. The costs of this procedure vary but are generally in the $300 to $700 range.

- *Dentist-supervised home bleaching:* The dentist first cleans your teeth and then takes impressions from which will be made a thin, clear plastic appliance (tray) that fits over your teeth. At home you fill the tray with a small band of gel that contains from 10 to 22 percent carbide peroxide and wear it from two to eight hours a day. The process can lighten teeth up to eight shades within a month. A touch-up is usually a good idea after two years. Again, costs vary and can range from $500 to $1,000—depending on the dentist.

- *Over-the-counter bleaching systems:* These are kits that can be purchased in the supermarket or drugstore, and they work in the same way as the dentist-administered trays. The difference is in the plastic forms in which the gel is placed. Sometimes the gel is not as effective and, without dental monitoring, it's possible for bleach to enter cracks in the teeth, eventually causing injury to the teeth.

Bleaching strips are new on the market, first put out in 2001 by Crest. These strips, which contain peroxide gel, are placed over the teeth twice a day for twenty minutes at a time. The results appear to be successful, but how long the good results last has yet to be determined. Currently, the price of such kits is under $50.

SMILE DESIGN

Dr. Rosenthal has a philosophy about what makes a beautiful smile. He calls it the *smile stage.* "We design a smile for patients according to their facial structure, skin tone, hair color, gender, and age," Rosenthal says. "The smile stage is not just teeth. It includes the lower third of the face. It is the raising of the *curtain* of the smile, which is the lips, and it includes the *scenery*, which is the gums, and the *actors*, which are the teeth. If you have a very gummy smile, that means that the curtain is probably too high, and so the actors are too small or the scenery is too big. Or both. It doesn't work. If your curtain is too heavy, which happens as you age, the upper lip drops from a loss of elasticity, and you cannot see the 'scenery' or the 'actors,' so you have to shorten the curtain a bit or lift it up.

"Tending to all these factors," says Dr. Rosenthal, "is what I call *smile design.* It includes a good look at the color, shape, size, and placement of the veneers or crowns. You want white, not *blindingly* white. The color has to relate to your eyes, hair, and skin tone." The shape of your teeth also should conform to the shape of your face. For example, longer teeth make a round face slimmer. A slim face requires wider teeth and a wider arch to make the face look better, the same way stripes going down vertically make you look thinner and horizontal stripes make you look heavier. The support of the lips and the lower third of the face come directly from the teeth. By building out a porcelain veneer, the facial area around the mouth is gently raised, thereby smoothing upper lip wrinkles, causing lips to appear fuller and poutier.

Tissue Recontouring

Attending to the gums is an alternative way to make a smile look better. Today, thanks to the diode laser, dentists can actually literally shape the gums in a matter of seconds. If someone has a "gummy smile," tissue can be moved into different positions to correct it. It used to take a full surgical procedure with stitches and waiting up to four to six weeks to heal. Today dentists can shape the gums with no bleeding, no pain, no trauma, and you look great immediately, with little downtime.

Lasers

Lasers continue to astound in their capacity to do marvelous things in dentistry. While the diode laser recontours tissue, the argon laser cures and sets the newest dental materials. For that reason dentists have a tremendous amount of time to manipulate the materials. When they are satisfied with the shape and position of the material, they cure it with the argon laser for five or ten seconds. Now they're working on a new type of erbium YAG laser with water that will actually cut hard tissue, which means—this is great news—instead of drilling, dentists will be able to cut into our teeth with no pain and no noise.

The dental revolution that began in the 1970s has taken the profession to new heights. As we enter the twenty-first century, dentistry will have even greater state-of-the-art materials, greater techniques, and more qualified dentists to deliver these services. At the center of all this is the patient, who will be on the receiving end of a less invasive, more predictable, and more naturally beautiful smile. It's as simple as one, two, three trips to your dentist.

AUTHORS' NOTE: We are particularly grateful for his assistance to Dr. Larry Rosenthal, a New York–based cosmetic dentist who has gloriously created and/or revitalized smiles in New York and the surrounding planet for the past twenty-five years. Dr. Rosenthal is the director of the Aesthetic Advantage Institute in Palm Beach, Florida, a teaching institution. He is also director of the Larry Rosenthal Institute for Aesthetic Dentistry at New York University.

twelve

The Nutrition/ Complexion Connection

Healthy skin does a lot more than look great. It sustains moisture throughout your body and sweats out "the bad stuff." But even skin in perfect condition needs constant protection and maintenance. That's because tiny molecules called *free radicals* attack our cells with regularity and eventually break them down. This cell breakdown is responsible for aging and, in some cases, even premature aging. It affects the tone and suppleness of our skin, and it affects collagen, the fibrous network that keeps skin plump and line-free. The result is the dermatological equivalent of corrosion. But take heart. Powerful chemicals known as *antioxidants* may help fight that corrosion. And because antioxidants can be found in so many of the foods available to us, if we eat the right things, we can literally fight the effects of aging with every bite.

Jane Brody, health columnist for the *New York Times*, wrote in a recent column on healthy eating, "It's not chronological but biological age that determines what you can and cannot do and I'm happy to report, it's biological aging that we have the potential to slow." In other words, by taking preventive measures now, we can reduce the chances of unnecessary damage to our complexions in the future.

To understand what these preventive measures are, we must first understand what causes aging in our cells in the first place. Follow me back to biology and chemistry class again for just a moment, if you will, as I try to explain the interaction between free radicals and their nemesis: anti-oxidants.

FREE RADICALS

Free radicals is a term you may have come across in the past ten years. A free radical is an atom or a molecule with an unpaired electron. Normally electrons come in pairs, so unpaired electrons make for highly unstable molecules. This unpaired electron in a free radical sends it charging into other molecules so it can "steal" an electron from them, which damages the other molecules and changes their structure, causing them to also become free radicals. This can create a self-perpetuating chain reaction, which, in the end, wreaks havoc with our DNA, protein molecules, enzymes, and cells.

Our skin is made up of cells. Each cell has a fatty layer that protects it. It's that fatty layer that is so susceptible to the free radicals. Free radicals, if given the opportunity, love to move in on the fatty layer (the receptor) of the cell. Once the free radical permeates the cell membrane, it changes the chemical structure of the cell itself, leading to cell break-down, which causes aging. But it's not just aging that free radicals encourage. Scientific research has shown that uncontrolled free-radical activity in the body is directly associated with a number of health problems, including the skin-related age spots, circulation problems, dry skin, varicose veins, and wrinkles.

Common external sources of free radicals are cigarette smoke, pollution, pesticides, herbicides, overexposure to the sun, automobile exhaust, and more. In our bodies they arise as a natural by-product of normal metabolic functions, such as in the detoxification processes and in our immune system defense. They also can be found in the food we eat, in our water supplies, and in the air we breathe. In other words, they're just about everywhere. But take heart. Help is just a bite away.

ANTIOXIDANTS

Antioxidants are the lead defenses in controlling or elimi-nating free radicals in the body. Antioxidants are natural compounds that act as scavengers, roaming the body look-ing for free radicals. They actually *protect* the cell membrane by forming a barrier so that the free radicals can't permeate it and essentially neutralize free radicals by donating one of their own electrons, ending the electron-stealing reaction.

Where foods come in is that certain foods contain specific types of antioxidants. It's important to understand the role these foods play in skin care and aging prevention. Which ones are highest in antioxidant content? The important antioxidants that we know about are vitamins A, C, and E. The B-complex vitamins also have a high antioxidant content. And as we shall see, minerals have a protective purpose as well.

Vitamin A

Vitamin A is an antioxidant with many roles, one of which basically is to prevent dry, scaly skin. If you have a sufficient amount of vitamin A in your diet, your skin will stay smoother and suppler. It can also help with wrinkles, because, as we know, dry skin wrinkles more easily than moist, supple skin.

Vitamin A comes in two forms: pure vitamin A and beta-carotene. *Beta-carotene* is not vitamin A per se, but when it is taken into the body, it gets converted into the active form of vitamin A. Foods rich in beta-carotene are plant-based. It's found in dark leafy green vegetables, including broccoli, spinach, and kale. It's also found in the yellow-orange foods, like cantaloupe, apricots, squash, pumpkin, carrots, sweet potatoes, and winter squash. One of the other sources is retinal, which can be converted to vitamin A in our bodies. These other sources come from animal-based foods, such as eggs, milk, cheese, dairy products, and liver. Our own liver actually stores a lot of pure vitamin A, as do the livers of animals. So any kind of liver is always an excellent source of vitamin A.

But beware. You can actually overdose on vitamin A. Vitamin A is a fat-soluble vitamin, which is stored in the liver, so it is not easily excreted—whereas water-soluble vitamins are excreted in the urine. Beta-carotene, which doesn't have the same toxic effect, gets stored just beneath the skin. The symptom of an overdose of beta-carotene is an orange-yellow tone to your skin. A large part of vitamin A in our diets comes from animal products, but these, as you know, can be high in cholesterol and fat. A well-balanced diet is always the best, and that means a combination of fruits and vegetables along with any animal products.

Vitamin E

Another big antioxidant is vitamin E, which is the most abundant fat-soluble antioxidant in the body and one of the most efficient antioxidants available. Vitamin E protects the cells from premature aging because it provides a barrier along the cell membrane, warding off the attack of free radicals. Remember that the cell membrane is a fatty lipid layer. Because vitamin E is fat-soluble, it strengthens and protects the cell by creating this barrier. It is also thought to protect against UV damage and to help preserve skin elasticity.

Vitamin E is usually found in whole, unprocessed grains, such as wheat, barley, rye, and wheat germ. Canola, sunflower, and safflower oils and many nuts such as hazelnuts and almonds are good sources. Soy, whether it's in its original form (edamame) or transformed into tofu, is loaded with vitamin E, which boosts new cell growth and keeps skin moist.

Basically, if you have a variety of these foods in your diet, you won't need a supplement of vitamin E. Most people get more than 100 percent of their RDA of vitamins A and E quite easily from their diets.

Vitamin C

Everyone has heard about vitamin C's helping to cure the common cold by boosting the immune system, but not many know that vitamin C is the most abundant water-soluble antioxidant in the body. It acts primarily in cellular fluid and is thought to combat free-radical formation caused by pollution and cigarette smoke. It is also helpful with the production and synthesis of elastin and collagen. Collagen gives skin its tone. Elastin promotes skin strength and elasticity in blood vessel walls and cell membranes. Vitamin C also helps with the metabolism of amino acids, which are the building blocks of all cells. The skin is composed of amino acids, so nourishment from vitamin C helps in the process of healing wounds, sores, or cuts.

Vitamin C is commonly found in fruits, most citrus fruits, and vegetables. Red, orange, and yellow fruits—oranges, mangoes, papayas, cantaloupes, and strawberries—tend to be high in vitamin C. Dark green vegetables such as spinach and green peppers are excellent sources as well. A hefty handful of strawberries has all the antioxidant vitamin C your body requires each day to reconstruct your collagen.

Vitamin B and B Complex

B complex is an extended group that includes B_1 and B_2 (thiamine and riboflavin), niacin, B_{12} and B_6. B complex is found in most foods that we eat, because most foods in the United States have to be fortified. So any grain food is fortified with B complex and B vitamins. Whole-grain foods—

like wheat, barley, rye, and wheat germ—are also full of B-complex vitamins. So are dark leafy green vegetables like spinach and broccoli.

Basically B vitamins help with skin color and tone. A deficiency of B vitamins can actually promote skin sores, cracked lips, and cracking at the corners of the mouth. Most of the Bs are used for energy production, and B_1 and B_2 are especially used for energy production within the cells. A deficiency of these can actually cause dermatitis, dry itchy, scaly, rashy skin.

B_{12} is found mostly in animal products, meat, fish, poultry, dairy products, and eggs. It actually helps with iron absorption and prevents anemia, a lack of iron in the blood that causes pale skin, fatigue, and loss of appetite. The body makes B_{12}; you don't have to take it as a supplement. It's involved in the development of rapidly dividing cells. Some of the cells in the body turn over very quickly, including the cells in your skin. They need the B vitamins for energy to help with that rapid turnover process.

Folate

Folate, another B vitamin, is found in dark leafy green vegetables, beans, and legumes as well as in liver. Folate is involved with the production of rapidly dividing cells, so it also helps with skin health. We shed the top layer of our skin every few weeks. The new skin that comes up is not going to be healthy skin unless you nourish your body from the inside, which is why folate is so important.

Flavonoids

Two antioxidants that are not commonly talked about are types of *flavonoids*. Flavonoids, which are plant pigments, have been found recently to have antioxidant effects. They give plants, trees, vegetables, and flowers their distinctive colors. Scientists have found that these flavonoids protect the plants against environmental stress, so they think that flavonoids, if ingested, may also do the same thing for us. Basically there are two types of flavonoids that have actual benefits. One is called *polyphenols*, which can be found, among other places, in green tea. These polyphenols in green tea may actually help in skin protection, and it has been found that these components, along with some other elements in green tea, may also have antiviral and anticarcinogenic effects. Berries are a great source of polyphenols as well. These fruits are currently being studied for their antiaging properties. The other type of flavonoids is called *proanthocyanins*. These are found in grapes and in pine bark. Not much research has been done, but it is under way, and hopefully we will soon know better what the direct connection is between these flavonoids and healthy skin.

Niacin

Niacin basically is another B vitamin found in whole-grain products and enriched grain products. Niacin is used in energy metabolism as well as to help support skin production, the nervous system, and digestion. A deficiency of niacin can cause dermatitis, which is an irritation of the skin, and rashes.

Minerals

Minerals, such as zinc and iron, are equally essential to having your skin be the best it can be.

ZINC

Zinc is a well-known antioxidant, essential for normal cell growth and repair. It can be found in whole grains, meat, most seafood, and onions. Zinc is involved in many enzymatic reactions. (Enzymes help to facilitate a chemical reaction.) It helps with protein synthesis and the production of skin cells and muscles. As good as it is, zinc can be toxic, so supplements are not recommended without a physician's direction. Taking more than two grams of zinc a day can produce the side effects of vomiting and diarrhea and can accelerate the process of atherosclerosis.

IRON

Iron helps to make red blood cells, and it helps the blood to carry oxygen to all the cells of the body, so if you are iron-deficient, you may not be providing your body with enough oxygen. As a result, the skin is pale, and the nails may become concave and spoon-shaped. Iron is found in animal products and in dairy products, but it's not always bioavailable—that is, the minerals from these foods are not readily absorbed by the body. Good sources of iron are red meat, fish, and chicken, as well as beans and spinach. Liver is the food highest in iron, because the liver is the organ that processes iron.

Protein

Protein is important for the production of muscle and skin cells. Whenever our cells regenerate—whether they're skin, muscle, or bone cells—they require protein. Very strict vegetarians may have difficulty getting enough protein, but they can complement it in other ways. What does this mean? Foods that come from animal products are considered complete protein. Foods that come from plant-based products are incomplete protein. So if you are not eating animal products, it becomes necessary to combine different types of plant products in order to get sufficient protein. Animal products have essential amino acids, which, as we have seen earlier, are what our bodies need to build or repair tissue. In plants you have to combine different things in order to get the full complement of essential amino acids. In other words, rice and beans, or different types of whole grains with nuts and seeds, taken together, will provide you with complete protein.

AUTHORS' NOTE: We greatly appreciate the gracious generosity of time and assistance with this chapter from Siri Sirichanvimol, M.S., R.D., Clinical Nutrition Manager at New York University Medical Center in New York City.

thirteen

Do Try This at Home

Up to this point, my role has been to show you what it takes to obtain beautiful, radiant, healthy skin. But my philosophy for looking terrific also incorporates how you *feel* about yourself—how confident you are when you leave your home each morning, ready to take on the world. None of what I've written so far works if you don't *feel* as if you look great.

Let's start with the realities: Everyone has natural beauty. Your mother told you that, and she was right. A pretty face is a unique face, a natural face. *Your* face. It's not the perfection of a supermodel. There *is* no perfect supermodel. Supermodels get blemishes, just as you and I do. Believe me. I treat them all the time. In addition, many of them—most of them—have uneven or imperfect features. Look at Lauren Hutton's smile. Look at any of these people without makeup and see how much they look like everyone else you pass on the street. What supermodels have is *confidence*, pure and simple. These people look great because they *think* they look great. No, they *know* they look great.

You may be wondering how you, too, can ooze confidence from every pore when you have a nose you hate and eyes that are too close together. What I say to that is: instead of focusing on what you *don't* have, focus on what you *do* have. Why not aim your sights at gloriously radiant, healthy skin—which, after reading this book, you now know how to achieve? If you're not there just yet, though, and if you can't forgive a feature or two, there's always the power of a little bit of camouflage. However, just a little bit. Imperfections at times are, well, perfection.

Here's what I think: Makeup as an enhancement is good. Makeup as camouflage is not. Makeup to conceal is good. Hiding is bad. Obliterating your natural skin tones with tons of makeup turns you into somebody else. If you have blemishes or wrinkles, you can safely conceal them, up to a certain point, but it's better always to get rid of the blemish, the imperfection, the brown spot, the blood vessel, or the wrinkle. Sometimes hiding something ends up making it look worse than before. Sometimes the more you hide, the more you see.

The first words most perceptive women say to their makeup artist are: "I don't want to look as if I'm wearing makeup." I couldn't agree more. If you have beautiful skin, why not flaunt it? If you don't—and I assume that if you're reading this book, you need at least some help—there are still many, many ways to look natural yet stunning. Read on. It's all about face.

THE EYES AND EYE MAKEUP

I am going to start with the eyes because I see them as the center of the cosmetic universe. If your eyes are glowing and glorious, most imperfections will pale by comparison. Eyes are easy. If you think about it, unlike every other feature on your face, your eyes don't age. Around the eyes, yes, but not your eyes per se. Still, if you're anyone other than Elizabeth Taylor, even the eyes can sometimes use a bit of help.

Selecting Eye Makeup

- All eye shadows should be in neutral hues. No matter what color your eyes are, leave the bright colors to the Las Vegas showgirls.

- Iridescent eye shadow is for teenagers. Period. Anything shiny in a cosmetic tends to collect in the creases, especially on your eyes.

Applying Eye Makeup

- For eyes too close together, apply a neutral shadow to the inner third of the eye and a deeper, though still neutral, color on the outer two-thirds. Start eyeliner about a third of the way out from the nose. Highlight beneath the upper-outer brow (along the brow bone) to visually widen the eyes.

- For eyes that are too wide apart, use deep to natural shades in the first third of the eyelid and go lighter as you blend out. Apply eyeliner to the first third of the eyelid only.

- For deep-set eyes, apply neutral to pastel shades on the lower lid area and avoid using deep, dark eyeliners.

- Puffy eyes require a slightly darker shade of foundation applied directly to the puffy area above the eye (see "Concealer" tips on page 224 for below the eye). Blend and set with a fine dusting of powder.

- Curling eyelashes opens the eyes.

- To make eyes appear bigger, apply a little bit of shimmer in the inside corner of the eyes.

EYEBROWS

Balance and a natural look are what well-shaped eyebrows bring to the face.

- Pluck brows in a room with plentiful daylight and using good tweezers. Pluck brows after a shower, when your pores are still open.

- Keep the beginning of the brow even with the inside corner of your eye. The rule along the length of the brow is to pluck only from beneath the brow. Let the brow extend beyond the outside corner of your eye. At that point it should taper slightly down.

- To define thin brows, use a powder shadow with a firm slant brush and feather-in your brows to achieve the shape you want. Stick as close as possible to your natural brow line.

- Powders let you layer on the color, which provides a more natural look than the penciled-on brow.

- For a natural look, coordinate your brow color with the color of your hair.

FOUNDATION

The object of using foundation is to even out skin tone and to cover up broken capillaries and brown spots.

Selecting a Foundation

- Choose a formula that suits your desired finish and then simply try two to three of the closest skin shades at your jawline. The color that blends in with your complexion at the jaw is your ideal foundation shade.

- If possible, check the color in daylight before purchasing any foundation. Look for the nearest window in the shop or simply walk outside with a small mirror.

- Thick, heavy base tends to accent wrinkles.

- Add water or moisturizer to bottled bases that get too thick or where the color is too intense.

Applying Foundation

- For a light, sheer look, dampen the sponge before applying foundation.

- Use foundation all over your eyelids and powder with a clear dust before applying eye color. This helps to keep color truer, and it will last longer.

- Use foundation in the center of the face where it is needed and blend out to the edges for the sheerest possible coverage.

CONCEALER

Concealer, which is noticeably thicker than foundation, is used to cover blemishes, dark spots, dark circles beneath the eyes, and other problem areas too prominent to be hidden by foundation.

Selecting a Concealer

- Concealers come in sticks, creams, and tubes. Select the one that is lightest in "feel" but still gets the job done.

- Avoid the impulse to choose a concealer that is too light in "color" when correcting under-eye darkness.

Applying Concealer

- Minimize bluish/violet under-eye circles by applying a yellow-based concealer, directly on top of the area. White concealer is going to make black circles appear gray.

- Always apply concealer directly to discolored areas and then apply a foundation to balance the color.

- For deep discolorations on the skin, blend concealer well into the skin, then apply foundation, and then put a bit of concealer on top of the foundation as well. For best results, use your fingertips.

- Always apply concealer to the dark area in the inside corner of the eye.

- For covering blemishes, take a little brush, spot the blemish with the brush, patting foundation over the concealer, and then set with pressed powder.

BLUSH

- Apply in a few light touches on the "apples" of your cheeks, sweeping up toward the brows and blending into the hairline.

- Keep blush sheer to blend with skin tones. Stay with natural earth-tone colors, avoiding reds and oranges.

- If you use bronzing powder, concentrate it on the cheeks, the forehead, the edge of the chin, and a little bit of a light dusting across the nose, which is where the sun would hit the skin.

CONTOUR POWDER

- To soften the contours of the face or to hollow the cheeks or to adjust the shape and length of the nose and chin, blend contour powder with a big brush onto the sides of the nose and a bit on the tip of the nose.

- Rosy or amber tones or anything in nude shades look best.

- Use a shade darker than your foundation but not so dark as to be noticeable.

- Do the same thing in the hollows of your cheeks and along the bottom of the jawline if you have a fuller face. This will bring definition to the face.

LIPS AND LIPSTICK

- To hide the signs of aging around the lips, first use a nude lip pencil drawn a little bit farther than your natural lip line. Then apply lipstick with a lip brush, which helps it stay put and will help you precisely place the lipstick so it doesn't move into the fine lines. This also helps to achieve the look of fuller lips.

- For extra staying power, blot the first application of lipstick, apply powder, and reapply your lipstick.

- To achieve fuller lips, use a concealer in the lip area and then apply the pencil. Extend and shape the mouth so it's correct and then apply the lipstick.

- Always choose a lip liner that matches your lip color.

- Matte-finish and "long-wearing" lipsticks can be drying. Creamy formulas are much more flattering.

- Choose a natural or light shade of lip gloss and apply it in the middle of your lips for a pouty look.

BLEND, BLEND, BLEND!

Never just apply makeup and leave it there. Always blend, blot, or brush everything. No makeup can look beautiful unless it is blended. Color that just sits on the skin is too harsh and unnatural. Obvious demarcations between colors look heavy-handed. You must blend, every step along the way, whether you do it with your finger or with a brush. It is very natural to put color on and "rub it in." You probably think you've been blending since the first moment you used makeup. Blending is a special art that allows you to create light and dark naturally. You should never create a dark shadow without highlighting.

HAIR MATTERS

You want a simple, clean, classic hairstyle that works with the shape of your face. Part of looking younger is having the right hairstyle, an *age-appropriate* hairstyle. One of the most aging mistakes in the world is to be fifty or sixty and have a hairstyle that's becoming on teenagers. A proper hairstyle as well as the proper hair color can make you look younger, better, and more natural.

If you have thinning hair, you want your hairstyle to conceal the problem. Growing your hair long in order to "look as if" you have more hair doesn't work. The longer your hair is, the more it pulls down, and the worse it looks. Shorter hair provides the look of more volume. Washing thinning hair every day is perfectly fine, too. It doesn't make the hair fall out, doesn't make it thinner, doesn't do anything bad. In fact, as your hair gets oilier, it becomes more matted down and looks thin even if it is not. Everyday washing is actually very good for your hair. Blow-drying does not hurt thinning hair either. In fact, you can do whatever you want, and it is not going to affect the thickness of your hair. The only things I don't suggest are a tight ponytail or cornrow braiding. The pressure on the hair follicle on a constant basis for many years can kill the hair follicle and may cause fraction alopecia, a form of hair loss.

Know your hair type and work with it. If your hair is fine to normal, look for products that provide body, shampoos with polymers and proteins and amino acids. Normal to coarse hair does well with products containing lanolin, oil, and methicone.

If you're getting a few gray hairs (or a lot), and if *au naturel* is not for you, the color you select can add years to your face or subtract years from it. Cover gray with a shade slightly lighter than your natural color. Lighter near your face makes you look younger and more radiant. Too dark can give the appearance of harsh and older. Men, this goes for you, too. I have perfectly white hair and have been this way since my midforties—but I'm blessed with all the hair I started with. However, because I have pale skin and white hair, to keep from looking washed out, I use just the slightest bit of a self-tanner on my face, when I remember, for contrast. (See, no secrets here.)

In summary, keep your hairstyle up-to-date, keep the color close to natural, and know that as you age, soft, light colors work better than starkly dark. For thinning hair, keep it short, clean, and then forget about it.

fourteen

Finding "Dr. Right"

This will be the shortest, though perhaps the most important, chapter in this book. If you plan to go to a cosmetic dermatologist, it is essential that you find the best one you possibly can. There are very few requirements for selecting that person, but all of them are measurably important; none is up for compromise.

Just for the record, here is the difference between a cosmetic dermatologist and a general dermatologist: A dermatologist is a physician who diagnoses and treats the skin for all types of disease. Some dermatologists have chosen to subspecialize in cosmetic dermatology, which means that in addition to, or instead of, treating diseases of the skin, they do cosmetic procedures such as those covered in this book. Hence, the name *cosmetic* dermatologist.

Understand that that is the only difference between the two.

Finding "Dr. Right"

When choosing a cosmetic dermatologist, the object is to find one who is artistic as well as scientific. All doctors have the same training, the same instruments, and access to the same technology. But in the end, only 20 percent of cosmetic dermatology is true science. The other 80 percent involves the skill, artistry, and experience of the physician. How do you separate the artist from the technician? I don't have the perfect answer. But here are a few dos and don'ts that should be helpful.

First, and I think most essential, is to try to go to somebody with whom a friend or relative has had experience—someone whose work you can see firsthand and you like. Then check that person's credentials. See how long he or she has been in practice. Ask the doctor, or a staff member, what kinds of lasers are used, whether the doctor owns the lasers, and what kinds of procedures he or she does. If the answer is that the doctor only does one kinds of procedure—Botox, for example—or rents the laser, he or she doesn't have the experience you need. Avoid this person at all costs. I mean it.

It's nice if you find the doctor to be a pleasant sort, but remember, chemistry is not always important. Oftentimes the best "personality" is not the best doctor. This is your face and your body we're talking about! What you need is someone with unquestionable skill; if that person also makes you laugh, more power to him or her.

CAVEAT EMPTOR

The question we've all been trained to ask before selecting a physician is, Are you board-certified? When you ask that question of the person about to peel your face and he or she says yes, ask in what specialty. The doctor had better not say "cosmetic dermatology," because *there is not as of yet any board certification for this specialty.* Dermatology, yes. But not cosmetic dermatology. People out there are doing lasers, and yes, they're board-certified, but they're board-certified in other specialties. I'll say this again. *There is no licensing facility—there's no board facility that controls the cosmetic world today.* None. Unfortunately.

So, how to find the right physician for you? Here is my answer, in a nutshell: In the best of all possible worlds, the physician you select must be well trained in dermatology, so at least you know he or she understands the functions of the skin and the anatomy. That person should be a *cosmetic* dermatologist who does a good number of procedures each week and owns the laser that is used. Finally, I think it is best if you know someone who has been to this doctor and you like the results you see. If you have no friends who have had these procedures (although it's more than likely that some of your friends have had these procedures but don't talk about them), ask for a recommendation from your family physician—but only if he or she knows the *work*, not just the doctor.

Epilogue

The great American philosopher Billy Crystal once said, "It's better to *look* good than to *feel* good." Well, *I* say, why not do *both*?

It's no secret. When you look better, you *feel* better. When you look more youthful, you *feel* more youthful. If a little bit of aging has replaced that fresh, dewy look with sallow skin or left wrinkles across your forehead and your upper lip, you're not going to feel sexy. Well, cheer up. Time may be marching on, but fortunately, technology is jogging along even faster.

As you have just seen, today's cosmetic dermatologist has an arsenal of antidotes for aging—antidotes that don't require surgery. We can polish and buff your skin with lasers that also hide imperfections such as age spots and spider veins. We can rebuild your collagen, which is responsible for 80 percent of your skin's foundation. We can fill in deep lines and scars with silicone, slough off dead skin with peels. Brighten and reshape your smile, transplant your hair or remove it. Today you can eat not only to *win* but also to boost your cells so they can defend themselves against attack.

But make no mistake. Skin rejuvenation is not only a scientific discipline. It is an evolving art as well. In this high-tech world of cosmetic dermatology, one can go too far. There is a level at which, instead of looking good, rested, naturally younger, you start looking fake, plastic, older. All cosmetic dermatologists have Botox, lasers, silicone, collagen; we all have the fillers and the removers. The art in this profession is knowing how much to do, when to do it, where to do it, and most important, when to stop. Eventually even the artist must put down his brush and declare his work finished.

A word about history. I still find it astonishing how very few of the medications, processes, and procedures mentioned in this book were in use ten years ago. And how much of what we now know about foods, and even exercise, has been learned recently. Think 1990. Who but the scientific types at that lofty Rockefeller University could sit over a cup of coffee and discuss free radicals? When did the term *glycolic acid* slip into the vocabulary of mainstream America? It has been an exciting decade, and certainly, within the next few years, materials we have not even dreamed of will be available, all in the name of beauty.

If this book has done nothing more, I hope it has delivered the following message: if you want to avoid plastic surgery but achieve comparable results, you need four things:

Epilogue

a well-trained dermatologist, a systematic approach, realistic expectations, and patience. Americans want quick fixes, but like anything good, rejuvenating your skin takes time, and it takes some work. In the end, though, I promise you, you are going to look marvelous. And because you will also look so *natural*, unless you tell them, your family and friends will never know what you've done.

But I'll bet you a vial of Botox, they'll be wondering.

Index

Index

hands, 122–31
heredity, 3, 15, 108, 134, 150
horse chestnut seed extract, 146
HQRA creams, 38–41
hyaluronic acid gel, 83–84, 186
hydration, 183–90
hydroquinone creams, 37–42
hyperpigmentation, 37
hypopigmentation, 36–37

I
iron, 217

K
keratinocytes, 13

L
L-ascorbic acid, 195
lactic acid, 191–92
laser facials, 65, 68
laser treatments. *See also* lasers
    advantages of, 4, 130
    choosing doctor for, 69–71
    how they work, 60–61
    nonablative, 68–69
    risks of, 27
lasers
    532 Medlite, 120, 130
    carbon dioxide, 62, 66–67
    erbium YAG, 62–68
    nonablative, 68–69
legs
    brown spots on, 144–45
    cellulite on, 95–96, 138–44
    conditioning, 145–47
    exercise for, 146–47
    healing times for, 144
    spider veins on, 134–38
    swollen, 146
    varicose veins on, 134–35, 137–38
light peels, 43–49
lines, 75, 76, 98, 172. *See also*
    wrinkles
liposuction, facial, 104–6
lips, sunscreen for, 183

lipstick, 116, 226–27
liquid nitrogen, 42
lotions, cleansing, 194–95

M
makeup, 116, 193–94, 220–27
massages, 141–43
medium-depth peels, 44, 49–50
melanin, 13, 36
men
    aging process in, 7, 171
    brown spots on, 172–73
    facial capillaries on, 173–74
    forehead lines on, 172
    hair loss in, 148–51, 153–58,
        165
    hair removal for, 100, 174–75
    in their fifties, 23
    in their forties, 21
    in their thirties, 19
    in their twenties, 18
mesotherapy, 4, 89–93, 95–96
microdermabrasion. *See*
    dermabrasion
microsuction, 104
millia, 190
minerals, 217
mini-liposuction, 126
minoxidil, 156–58
moisturizers, 115, 176, 181, 183–88

N
N-Lite lasers, 68–69
necks, 75, 101–2
niacin, 216
nose, shaping, 102
nose, veins near, 173–74
nourishing skin, 192–96
nutrition
    antioxidants, 195, 212–18
    free radicals, 209, 210–11

O
oil glands, 13–14, 192–93
ointments, cleansing, 194–95

Index